HYSTERIA, HYPNOSIS AND HEALING
THE WORK OF J.-M. CHARCOT

Books by A. R. G. Owen :

Can We Explain the Poltergeist?
Science and the Spook. (With *Victor Sims*)

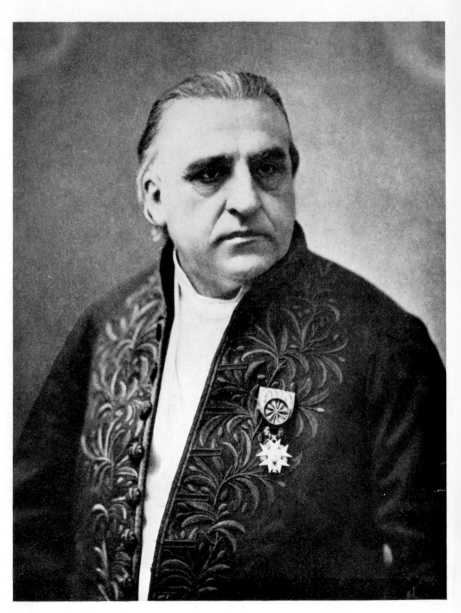

Jean-Martin Charcot

A. R. G. Owen

HYSTERIA, HYPNOSIS AND HEALING THE WORK OF J.-M. CHARCOT

LONDON : DENNIS DOBSON

ISBN 0 234 77455 X

First published in 1971 by
Dobson Books Ltd., 80 Kensington Church Street, London W.8

Printed in Great Britain by
Bristol Typesetting Co. Ltd., Bristol 2.

To
EILEEN GARRETT
who
like Charcot always searched
for the truth wherever it might
be found.

CONTENTS

Chapter		*Page*
	Preface	XI
I	Ancient and Modern Medicine	13
II	The Founder of Neurology	29
III	The Discovery of the Neuroses	55
IV	The Causes of Hysteria	85
V	Cure, Faith, and Healing	124
VI	Metals and Magnets	147
VII	Hypnotism before Charcot	170
VIII	Hypnotism at the Salpêtrière	184
IX	Charcot and the Supernatural	212
X	Citizen Charcot	217
	References	235
	Appendix	247

ILLUSTRATIONS

Jean-Martin Charcot   *Frontispiece*
  (*Courtesy Radio Times, Hulton Picture Library*)

The Hospital of the Salpêtrière   *facing page* 32
  (*Courtesy Radio Times, Hulton Picture Library*)

Charcot in 1848 when promoted Internat des Hôpitaux.
Portrait in l'Hôpital de la Charité.   33
  (*Courtesy Masson et Cie, Paris*)

Charcot examining a brain. From a 1875 sketch by Brissaud.   64
  (*Courtesy Masson et Cie, Paris*)

Demonstrating hysteria.   65

Justine Etchverry, subject of 'traumatic neurosis', hysterical
  ischuria, and a 'miraculous cure', by suggestion.
Hysterical attack in 'traumatic neurosis'.   74
  (From *Clinical Lectures I*)

Hysterical contracture of the left hand.
Experiment intended to certify the reality of the contraction
of the hand.   75
  (From *Clinical Lectures III*)

Hysterogenic zones on the front of the body
Arrangement of the apparatus in the experiments on
catalyeptic immobility.   90
  (From *Clinical Lectures III*)

Anesthesia produced in successive stages, A, B, C by
  hypnotic suggestion (Case of Greuz-).
Hysterical anesthesia (Case of Porcz-).
Hysterical anesthesia (Case of Pin-).   91
  (From *Clinical Lectures III*)

PREFACE

MY INDEBTEDNESS to Professor Georges Guillain's invaluable study of Charcot's life and work, published first in 1955, is vast and will be obvious to any reader familiar with his book. Charcot has not been excessively exposed to the activities of biographers, but some explanation should be offered for attempting to supplement Professor Guillain's admirable study. Sufficient justification for this book lies, I hope, in its shift of emphasis. Professor Guillain, as a successor of Charcot's in the Chair of Clinical Diseases of the Nervous System in Paris, very naturally and properly stressed Charcot's work in physiology and neurology. Consequently his account of Charcot's investigations into the neuroses, hypnotism, and the psychology of suggestion and faith healing, though eminently accurate and fair, is necessarily somewhat brief and condensed.

Yet it so happens that in these latter topics there resides a world of interest for readers of the most diverse kinds: the medical student, the historian of science, the general practitioner of medicine, the educated layman who wishes to acquaint himself with the antecedents of psychoanalysis and the problems of the unconscious, and all those as well who desire a more precise knowledge of the somewhat 'occultist' topics—hypnotism, mesmerism, somnambulism, and faith healing. Although this book contains little 'parapsychology,' there is in its pages inevitably much of great relevance to parapsychology, and I hope that I have impartially conveyed general knowledge that will be useful alike to those interested in psychology as well as to those who are intrigued by the problems of psychical research.

It was through parapsychology that I became involved in the writing of this book. But I must confess that, at the outset, I had little inkling of the fascination and central importance of the problems studied by Charcot. Had it not been for Eileen Garrett's unique insight, the work would never have been undertaken; without her patient encouragement it would not have been completed.

A. R. G. Owen
Cambridge, 1969

CHAPTER 1

Ancient and Modern Medicine

JUST ONE hundred years ago, when a Napoleon was still Emperor of the French, a lecture was given in Paris entitled 'Empirical and Scientific Medicine; Comparison Between the Ancients and the Moderns.' The lecture was somewhat modestly presented, a mere introduction to a course on senile and chronic diseases. But it was delivered by a great man and was more than a trite occasional piece. It could serve equally well today as an introduction to many of the main issues in twentieth-century psychology, psychiatry, and parapsychology.

The opening words tell us much about the lecturer.

You now know the object of these studies : we might plunge directly into the subject for I am of Condillac's opinion, and think that general considerations are best placed at the end, than at the beginning of a course. But there exists a kind of classical tradition which obliges the professor first of all to explain himself, more or less categorically, on certain fundamental questions, and to declare, so to speak, his profession of scientific faith. . . .

There is a simple and, so to speak, natural means of approaching the larger questions : it is to examine how, in the course of the progressive development of scientific culture, such questions have arisen, and how they have been solved; history thus becomes a means of criticism. Now in following this method one soon perceives that at no period has pure observation succeeded in dominating the spirit of speculation without supreme efforts. As for Medicine . . . even the most stoical intellects have never been found to limit themselves to establishing facts without trying to connect them by some sort of theory : from the beginning we see minds occupied as much (or even more) with the subjective relations of things as with objective reality; newly acquired empirical observations are compared and tested with one another, in order to make theories or systems issue from them.

But the lecturer goes on to grant that

There lies a necessity of the human mind, and it seems, to use a celebrated expression of Kant's, that our thoughts are necessarily formed in this human mould. This was clearly recognized by the founder of the Positive Philosophy himself [Auguste Comte], and no one will reproach him with opening the door to hypotheses when he declared that, though a theory should be exclusively based on observations, it is absolutely necessary to be guided by a theory in order to devote oneself to observation fruitfully.

But we can always distinguish the real needs of our intellect from the exaggerations of every kind into which the lovers of systems allow themselves to be drawn. We recognize in fact the existence of a speculative method based rigorously upon facts, as well as the existence of a method of observation, which keeps itself as far as possible from premature speculations; and consequently we have now only to find out on what grounds these two methods can unite.[1]

The speaker was a man 'in the middle of life's journey,' yet already a professor (*Agrégé*) in the Faculty of Medicine. For five years, Dr Jean-Martin Charcot had been Physician to the Hospital of the Salpêtrière. He was already distinguished but his fame was meagre in proportion to what the next twenty years would bring, when the world would acknowledge him as the creator of a new science—modern neurology. After a century, though his reputation has been gnawed at by lesser men, his fame remains, and we can recognize in him the great clinician who gave an essential impulse to medical psychiatry and the discovery of the unconscious.

In 1867 Charcot's lectures were part of the official teaching of the Paris Medical Faculty, but they were given in an informal milieu, in a side ward or a kitchen converted into a lecture room which, though small, could accommodate his audience. Yet, as shown by the excerpt already quoted, Charcot's style, though direct and unpretentious, was anything but casual. His argument was calm and logical and, like everything he ever did or wrote, was both precise and illuminating.

Though Charcot represented this particular lecture as being merely an offering to the demands of convention, the lecture itself went deeper than this formal requirement. It is, in fact, a document marking a definite moment in the history of medical and biological thought. The year 1867 can be taken as conveniently as any other in the mid-nineteenth century to signify the coming of age of the physiological sciences. Much remained backward in general medical attitudes; numerous techniques awaited development; but the philosophy and basic method of biological and medical science were by then essentially the same as they are now. Thus Charcot could say that in his day medicine had seen a profound and radical revolution taking place. He himself was not only a prime representative of that revolution, but also the most aware and conscious of its agents and among the ablest exponents of its principles. Though the triumph of these principles had been deferred to the nineteenth century, Charcot discerned them as having been formulated in the remote past. We may be encouraged therefore to cast a glance at the shape of ancient medicine.

Four essentially different strands can be recognized in the curative procedures of the ancient world : (1) the religious, (2) the magical, (3) the empirical, and (4) the causal, that is, the analytical. It is not easy to disentangle these strands, for they tended to merge in different proportions in various bodies of practice. Thus folk medicine combines an assortment of methods based on very different premises. Indeed, the word *medicine* itself results from primitive practice, being named after Medea— the mother of witchcraft; that is to say, magic and the remains of primeval and proscribed religions. She was also the mistress of *pharmacon* or drugs, including not merely herbs and simples of empirically proven efficacy, but also magical potions whose power was supposed to derive not only from inherent properties but from the rites of preparation and the spells laid upon them. Not all 'simples' or 'home recipes,' of course, got into the pharmacopeia purely by empiricism. Many graduated on the basis of fortuitous religious connections, such as an association with a lunar goddess as in the case of willow bark, a specific for rheumatism.[2] Sometimes these recipes were valueless or harmful and had to wait until modern times before they were thrown out of the physician's repertoire. But on occasion a specific became certified as sound on the basis of continued experience, the original crazy reason for its adoption having been totally forgotten.

Professional medicine in the ancient empires doubtless grew out of folk experience, but as a result of its ancestry maintained much that was magical and nonsensical alongside a great deal that was soundly based. From the medical tablets in the great library at Nineveh accumulated by the imperial bookworm Assurbanipal, we see magical and empirical elements combined in the armory of the professional physician. The physician seems to have been distinct from the priest, although religious notions were still active in justifying many medical practices. Thus the use of water was highly recommended because it was the element of Ea, who was particularly respected as a healing god—perhaps justly so, as a patron of cleanliness and hygiene. Conversely, the commands of religion could be invoked to sanctify ordinances arrived at by enlightened empiricism, as in the code of public health and preventive medicine which in the Hebrew books of Leviticus and Deuteronomy were presented as proceeding from the Supreme Authority.

The numerous professional physicians of Egypt, highly regarded by the Greeks, were distinct from the priests and temple healers, but were expected to conform with the procedures indicated in the medical canon—six books out of the thiry-two treatises of the Hermetic corpus ascribed to the god Thoth. Folk or empirical recipes were well to the fore, with many fantastic and unsavory prescriptions. Yet the Egyptian physicians seem to have been good diagnosticians, and some items in their pharmacopeia are still in use, such as opium, saffron, and the oils of castor and olive. They had some sound ideas belonging to analytical medicine. Climate and the absorption of toxins were recognized as causative factors. But the advance of causal medicine was handicapped by the fatally erroneous theory, current in Egypt and Asia Minor, that numerous affections of mind and body resulted from demonic action or demonic possession of the patient. This belief was evident in the medical theory of Vedic India, but declined in later Indian medicine which, of all the ancient systems outside Greece, came nearest to the ideal condition of a medicine both empirical and causal.

Greek medicine is, of course, the most interesting of all to ourselves as lying in the direct ancestry of our own. If we leave out of account folk medicine and the practice of prayer to the gods in general, we find that Greek medical theory comprised three distinct schools or trends. Their co-existence and interaction were by no means fruitless, but their approaches differed fundamentally.

According to myth, Asclepios (or Aesculapius in Latin) was the child of Apollo and Coronis. When Artemis slew the latter, Apollo, with great presence of mind, performed a caesarean operation and put Aesculapius in the care of Chiron, the Centaur. The famous sage taught him the art of medicine, in which Aesculapius became so proficient that he raised many noted men from the dead, including the heroes Lycurgus and Tyndareus. On receipt of a complaint from Hades, Zeus struck Aesculapius dead, but restored him to life after Apollo had gone surety for his good behavior. This fulfilled a prophecy made by Chiron's daughter that Aesculapius would be a god, die and become a god again.[3]

This sequence seems an accurate reflection of the actual history of the Aesculapian myth. Some place the origin of the cult in Thessaly, or even in Egypt, but it may have originated at Aesculapius' best-known temple, the one at Epidauros in Argolis. The first shrine was doubtless that of a local earth-deity, the possessor of a sacred spring. When Apollo attained to general eminence the shrine, following normal practice, would officially be regarded as that of a dead hero—of a 'son' of Apollo's. Finally the popularity of his healing cult transformed the patron Aesculapius once again into a god.[4]

On arrival at an Aesculapian temple, the patient first took a course of ritual purification consisting of an austere dietary regimen, baths, and purgation (doubtless with hellebore, a time-honoured recipe going back to the sage Melampos, the legendary founder of Greek medicine). The period of preparation was followed by 'incubation.' For one or more nights, the patient would sleep in the temple waiting for a healing dream. When retiring at dusk, he would say prayers and make offerings. Quite often the awaited dream would come, and the patient would be questioned by the god. Perhaps suggestion was adequate to bring this about, because there is no evidence to support the view of some modern writers that dream inducing drugs or hypnosis were employed.[5] Others suppose that a priest disguised as the god perambulated in the night, bringing with him a serpent or a sacred dog.[6] The Aesculapian shrines contributed much to subsequent medicine. In addition to bequeathing the word *clinic*, they encouraged hygiene, rest, change of scene, and the principle of hospitalization. Vitruvius, writing *On Architecture* about 30 BC, recommends the choice of salubrious sites for Aesculapian clinics. Walter Pater gave a charming, though possibly idealized, description in his novel *Marius the Epicurean* of how we might imagine a Roman Aesculapian temple to have looked.

It is possible, as some suppose, that the alternative school of medicine—analytical and empirical—associated with the name of Hippocrates grew up in some degree of conjunction with the Aesculapian cults. At the clinics the physician could make comparative studies on many patients and develop a symptomatology, aided by the long lists of symptoms recorded on the walls of the temples. But the Hippocratic writers did not learn all their arts 'in temples by observing real or supposed supernatural intervention, but . . . by experience and the application of reason to the nature of men and things.'[7] The Hippocratic Corpus is a collection of writings going back to the fifth century BC.[8] It was copied and preserved in the library at Alexandria and possibly constituted the original library of the Hippocratic school in the island of Cos. Perhaps thirteen of the books can be ascribed to Hippocrates—the 'Father of Medicine'—himself. The tract *On Ancient Medicine* seems to have been written to combat the influence of 'philosophical medicine,' which was being developed in the Pythagorean settlements in Italy, and sought to deduce the principles of medicine from *a priori* philosophical and cosmological theories. The Hippocratic author traces the history of food production to show that reliable knowledge can only be reached by intelligent empiricism. He asserts that the causes of disease cannot be reduced to the play of a few abstractions such as the Empedoclean qualities : cold, dry, hot and wet. On the contrary, the causes of disease are many and various and must be looked for concretely in actual environmental conditions and in human physiology; that is, in the capacity of the organism to react to external factors. Medicine, says the author, is not a branch of philosophy but of practical art, *technè*, and if this is forgotten it is the patient who suffers.

The Hippocratic physician agreed with de Condillac and Charcot that general considerations come better at the end of a study than at the beginning. It was idle, he said, to deduce the causes of disease and choose a course of treatment by deciding at the outset, from some philosophical principle, what Man is. On the other hand, 'clear knowledge about the nature of man can be acquired from medicine and no other source.' By medicine the Hippocratic physician means the careful observational study of both the healthy and the sick and the use of logical deduction. Causes 'that cannot be observed by the eye or the ear ought to be tracked by reasoning' (*The Art*). Here we have, indeed, truly *causal medicine*, based on the ascertainment of actual causes by observation and deduction just as in the modern way, but existing as Charcot says, 'in a very distant time.' This is what Charcot called the 'speculative method based rigorously upon facts.' Similarly, the author of the Hippocratic *Precepts* would have agreed with Comte and Charcot that it is necessary to be guided by some sort of theory, 'in order to devote oneself to observation fruitfully,' for he says : 'Now I approve of theorizing if it lays its foundation in incident, and deduces its conclusions in accordance with phenomena.'

Aesculapian temples thrived for centuries, until at last the Christians closed them or converted them into churches. Though Hippocratic medicine continued to be practiced, its advance was limited, its peak of development being realized in Galen (AD 130-200), the physician to the Emperor Marcus Aurelius. Greco-Roman science suffered from two handicaps, distinct but not unrelated. Society tended ever more decisively toward the ideal sketched in Plato's *Laws*—the absolute state based on slavery.[9] Where manpower is abundant, technology languishes. The ancient aristocracy and merchant class thought, as did Xenophon (*ca.* 427-355 BC), of the mechanical arts as carrying 'a social stigma and rightly dishonored in the Greek cities.' The technological basis of scientific instrumentation was, therefore, never established in ancient times. The microscope, the stethoscope, and numerous other aids to investigation had to wait on techniques developed not in the Renaissance, but in the despised Middle Ages. With equally serious effect Plato had cast doubt on the possibility of valid scientific knowledge and had turned men's thoughts to an immortality mystically attained, rather than to the more mundane task of increasing the expectation of life. Even Galen's work was tainted with error derived from the philosophical approach to biology. As for Aesculapian medicine, it became more invaded by charlatanry, and the patients were beaten to expel the demons of sickness.[10]

Christianity therefore is not obliged to shoulder all the blame for the retreat from science. But even so, charity bids us pass over in silence the thirteen centuries from Galen to Vesalius. It is sufficient indictment to note that, when Vesalius wished to study anatomy, no better textbook than Galen's was available.

'I think I recognize the essential difference between ancient and modern medicine,' said Charcot in his lecture of 1867. The former 'has always wanted the elements necessary to build up a positive theory [i.e., the material instruments and techniques of scientific enquiry] and that is why the numerous attempts it made in that direction always came to grief.' He went on to say that now (in the mid-nineteenth century) 'The moderns on the contrary possess some of the materials which can be used in this work of construction, but above all they know, profiting by the errors of their predecessors, which roads ought to remain closed to speculation and which, on the contrary, they may traverse without fear of losing themselves.'[11]

Charcot saw medicine in his day as having gone through a radical and profound transformation. But the links of tradition were not broken. They reached back via Harvey and Vesalius to Galen and Hippocrates. An immense heritage was preserved, but new horizons opened up. The essential character of the revolution was the intervention of anatomy and physiology in the domain of pathology. Diseases were no longer treated purely descriptively as collections of symptoms incident to the patient. Instead, following the doctrine of Bichat (1771-1802), the founder of general anatomy, medicine had to be causal—searching for the seat of the trouble in the tissues and recognizing disease as a disturbance of the inherent properties of our organs. Charcot then enunciates a principle : 'We do not have to do with the appearance of fresh laws, but with the perversion and derangement of pre-existing laws.'[12] Here Charcot, wiser than many before and since his time, is formulating the modern credo of scientific biology and psychology which postulates the lawfulness of biological phenomena and asserts the possibility of real knowledge concerning them.

Charcot comments on the two extremist points of view which had only recently waned. On the one side lay *vitalism*, which—as Charcot neatly put it—'detached from the organism the principles of life in order to make them rule over it as capricious tyrants.'[13] Recalling that only twenty years earlier, German biology and medicine had been in a deplorable condition under the sway of Schelling's 'Philosophy of Nature,' which engendered a fashion of 'poetic' points of view and transcendental conceptions, Charcot did not regret the supersession of this philosophy by the analytical approach. On the other side were schools whose vice was an oversimplification which was, to say the least, premature. These were the precursors of the behaviorists and 'reductionalists' of latter days, and they tended to reduce man's mental and psychic attributes to the subordinate status of *epiphenomena*. The iatromechanists thought in terms of de La Mettrie's slogan 'Man a Machine'; the iatrochemists reduced everything to chemistry.[14] Charcot thought that to give a physical or chemical interpretation of life was a rash endeavor, but he felt at the time of speaking that causal medicine had become free from the peril of falling into the errors of either vitalism or mechanism.

In a memorable passage, Charcot defines with great care an attitude that was destined to be entirely representative of medical biology in the next hundred years :

Always remembering that living beings present phenomena which are not found in dead nature, and which consequently are their especial property, the new physiology absolutely refuses to consider life as a mysterious and supernatural influence which acts at the instigation of caprice and is free from every law.

It goes so far as to believe that vital properties will one day be combined with properties of a physical order : at least, it insists for the future that a correspondence not an antagonism, must exist between these two forms of energy.

It sets itself to reduce all the vital manifestations of a complex organism to the action of certain organs only, and this again to the properties of certain tissues, of certain well-defined elements.

It does not seek the ultimate nature, or the wherefore of things for experience has shown it that the human mind cannot go beyond the *how*, that is beyond the immediate causes or the conditions of existence of phenomena. It recognises that in this relation the limits of our knowledge are the same in biology as in physics and chemistry. It remembers that beyond a certain point, as Bacon said, Nature becomes deaf to our questions and replies to them no longer.[15]

Lastly Charcot reviews the actual technical developments of the preceding half-century which had made the prospects for analytical medicine hopeful. Pathological anatomy had been systematized as a result of the efforts of Frenchmen and had taught physicians to think anatomically. Physiology had been entirely renovated and entered on the path of experiment indicated by Magendie and Levallois and visualized 'the living active organ.' Furthermore, physiology penetrated below the superficial features 'into the depths of the organ'; it probed into the functional organization of the cell. This was being made possible through the new technique of microhistology, which tended more and more 'to be a study of the living tissue and to correlate with clinical observation.' Finally, the growth of biochemistry had enabled the search for derangements of function, that is, faults in metabolism and chemical organization that could constitute disease in the absence of any discernible structural or morphological sign.[16]

So much for the speaker and his scientific Weltanschauung.

What of the place he spoke in, the hospital of the Salpêtrière? Like Charcot himself, this institution occupies a unique place in the history of mental healing. In the decades subsequent to 1867, Charcot and the Salpêtrière became completely identified, and to this day can hardly be thought of apart. But a century ago the hospital was already famous in its own right. It already commemorated a moment in the history of psychiatry—indeed, in the history of Man. It symbolized a revolution in society's attitude toward the insane and a refutation of a faulty medical opinion that had reigned for one and a half millennia.

The early Greek view of mental illness was indolent and incurious. In the tradition of Homer, 'the Bible of the Greeks,' a man became insane because the gods had made him irrational; they took his wits away. Various crude remedies such as purgative hellebore were considered as possibly beneficial, but apart from this lowly empiricism there was only mystical prejudice except in the ranks of causal medicine. The Hippocratic author of *The Sacred Disease*, a treatise on convulsive attacks of an epileptiform nature, recognized only natural causes. Or rather, though it is clear to us that he put aside the 'supernatural' as irrelevant to science, he devised an ingenious formula, possibly to avoid charges of atheism or impiety :

This disease styled sacred comes from the same causes as others, from the things that come and go from the body, from cold, from sun and from the changing restlessness of winds. These things are divine. So that there is no need to put the disease in a special case and to consider it more divine than the others; they are all divine and all human. Each has a nature and a power of its own; none is hopeless or incapable of treatment.

Although Plato emphasized the gods as the givers of divine prophetic mania, a series of Greco-Roman medical writers maintained the naturalistic approach of the Hippocratics. Asclepiades, an Epicurean, who lived in the first century of the Christian era, had a startlingly modern view. He ascribed mental diseases to emotional disturbances and distinguished them from the toxic deliria occuring in fevers which—he maintained—were organically caused. Galen, on the other hand, advanced a purely

23

biochemical theory, which explained mental illness as due to an imbalance among the various fluids postulated as residing in the body : namely, the *animal spirits* and the four *humors*. But this, though fanciful and erroneous, was at least a naturalistic explanation.

But after Galen attitudes retrogressed like the declining Roman Empire itself. Folk medicine, superstitions, and charlatanry flooded back into the profitable practice of medicine. As Plutarch scornfully remarked in his *Life of Cato*, the liver of a dead athlete was a sovereign talisman against epilepsy. Galen, in his work *The Pulse*, ridiculed the followers of Moses and Christ as being so rigidly sectarian as to be unworthy of the name of physician or philosopher. Be this as it may, the fact remains that before long Christian Emperors had to pass numerous decrees against ubiquitous magical and superstitious arts, so strong was the general retreat to obscurantism among pagans and Christians alike. Many of the pagan authors ascribed mental illness to attack or invasion by spirits. Eventually it became the prevailing belief that the insane were so as a result of demonic infestation. Any attempt at medical cure being considered pointless, mental illness passed out of the realm of medicine and into the sphere of demonology and exorcism. In the eleventh-century encyclopedia written by Michael Psellus in Byzantium, the medical section was devoted entirely to the hierarchy of demons who disturb the working of the human soul.[17]

The practical outcome of this philosophy was that the insane or mentally disturbed suffered one or the other of various fates, all unsatisfactory. For the most part they were left to their families to be dealt with, and these were the most fortunate though doubtless they were exposed to various folk remedies. Only occasionally did a municipality or a religious community make special provision for the mentally sick. If they lacked relatives, or were abandoned by them, the mentally disturbed, as objects of ridicule or hostility, wandered about mainly at night, tending to hide during the day. Some of the milder cases were able, like some mental defectives, to subsist as beggars on pity and alms. But generally the healthy tended to shun the mentally afflicted as being the abodes of evil spirits and, under the influence of theology, were inclined to regard them as sinful

24

accomplices of these demons. The more excitable and violent among the mentally ill were treated according to a doctrine handed down through Celsus, the author (or redactor) of the first medical work written in Latin. This treatise (produced in the reign of Tiberius) is humane and enlightened, but advocates harsh corrective measures for all except mild cases and confinement for the violent, who ought to be chastised by 'hunger, chains and fetters.' Consequently, throughout the Middle Ages right into modern times, the insane were liable to be flogged and imprisoned with diet meagre, but fetters abundant and flogging repeated. Except for the beatings, such treatment tended to be applied even in the hostels attached to religious houses and to the various healing shrines such as that of St Dympna in Belgium who was revered as the healer and patron saint of the insane.[18]

Often enough the disturbed received additional and unofficial punishment by way of blows and ridicule from the derelicts and criminals often confined with them. The keepers made money from the public. Aldous Huxley quotes from the memoirs of Louise du Tranchay concerning her experiences when committed in 1674 to La Salpêtrière.[19] She was chained up in a cage for public entertainment, and the visitors would poke at her with walking sticks. When we recall that this was in the time of the learned and benign Colbert, it underlines the fact of 'the neglect and prejudice in relation to mental disorders which tend to persist as a continuing background.'[20] It was possible even in 1863 for Charles Reade, the Oxford scholar and novelist, to sketch in *Hard Cash* a lurid picture of the treatment of mental patients. As late as 1917, the great American physician Thomas Salmon felt it imperative to comment poignantly on the neglect of mental patients even in progressive and forward looking communities. 'It is only through the most prolonged effort in the face of passive resistance that the right of the insane to kindness and care has won to practical acceptance.'[21]

Of course, the movement toward proper treatment of the psychiatrically disturbed had its eminent representatives in the United States and England, as evidenced by the names of Rush and Tuke. But in this book we are developing the story only in respect of France, where the fate of the mentally ill is intimately bound up with that of the Salpêtrière. This great hospital is

25

situated in its own grounds of about a hundred acres on the left bank of the Seine near the Quai d'Austerlitz, the Jardin des Plantes, and the Gâre d'Orléans. It takes its name from the original group of buildings erected there during the reign of Louis XIII as a powder magazine and called the Petit Arsenal-Salpêtrière (Little Arsenal). During the Frondist insurrections work was interrupted, and some of the buildings fell into disrepair. When the civil strife had come to an end, Paris, like ancient Rome, was the haunt of beggars and poverty-stricken nomads who had flocked to the capital, occasioning both the efforts of charitable organizations and grave fears for public order. Leading the charitable movements in Paris was a very remarkable man, Saint Vincent de Paul. Even a church composed entirely of freethinkers might consider his canonization (in 1737) as justifiable merely in virtue of his words, 'Mental disease is no different to bodily disease, and Christ demanded of the humane and powerful to protect, and the skilful to relieve the one as well as the other.'

Cardinal Mazarin set up the Hospice Général in 1656 under the authority of Vincent de Paul. This was a state department of hospitals for the confinement of beggars, of the destitute, of derelict women, and of the infirm. Bicêtre was reserved for men, Scipion for expectant mothers, and the Salpêtrière for women and prostitutes. The Cardinal also constructed a new building at the Salpêtrière. In 1657, begging was prohibited, and all Parisian beggars were rounded up. By 1663, the Salpêtrière contained 3,000 persons; in the eighteenth century it had become by far the largest asylum in Europe, with a population of 8,000. It comprised a maternity ward; a nursery for foundlings; infirmaries for the aged, the mentally defective, the paralytic, and the chronically ill; and an almshouse for veterans and a workhouse for destitute women. In addition there was within its walls the 'second Bastille,' the famous prison La Force. The latter was adjoined by Les Loges des Folles, a primitive quarter of unsanitary cells reserved for demented women who were frequently fettered and attacked by rats.[22]

Though some improvements were made in the course of the eighteenth century, this uniquely fantastic fortress of misery, the result of a paradoxical unity of charitable concern and public callousness, remained essentially unchanged until the French Revolution. The Revolution derived in part from three centuries of critical thinking during which every compartment of knowledge came under analysis and reconstruction. Robert Boyle's *Sceptical Chymist* (1661) was matched by skeptical biologists and physicians, and the Hippocratic spirit was being reborn as scientific medicine. It is to the eternal honor of France that French physicians were the prime representatives of the new order in psychiatry. Thus Joseph Daquin 'understood that the treatment of insanity should be highly analogous to the methods used in the study of natural history,' and that one should 'rid oneself of all prejudice against insanity.' He dedicated the second edition of his *Philosophie de la Folie* to a younger contemporary, Philippe Pinel, whom he considered 'a true friend of mankind, a man of virtue and enlightenment, an able physician in all departments of the art of healing, especially in the thorny subject of mental diseases.'

Pinel, who was born in 1745, came to Paris as a young physician eleven years before the Revolution. A friend of Benjamin Franklin's, he had considered emigrating to the United States. As it was, Pinel became physician-in-chief of the Bicêtre hospital and the Salpêtrière, continuing so under the Convention, the Directory, the Empire, and the Restoration, until he died at the age of eighty-one in his living quarters at the Salpêtrière. An enlightened conservative, studious and learned, he did not attempt to be a politician. Devoted to medicine, he had a profound bias toward the scientific, the logical, and the clear-cut. Pinel first wrote on mental diseases in 1787. He was appointed to the Bicêtre in 1793 and immediately sought to relieve the occupants of that 'pandaemonium' less vast only than that of the Salpêtrière. An official went with Pinel to the Bicêtre and put the question : 'Are you mad yourself, Citizen, that you want to unchain these animals?' When Pinel declared his conviction that the mentally ill were agitated only because deprived of fresh air and liberty, he was told : 'You may do as you please!' Not long after, Pinel, whose moderateness as a revolutionary brought him under suspicion as a royalist, was saved from an angry crowd by Chevigné, a former soldier whom he had released after ten years in fetters.[23]

Pinel was given also the administration of the Salpêtrière. A painting hanging in the lecture theatre shows him at les Loges des Folles, supervising the striking off of the chains—a symbolic event reversing attitudes maintained through two millennia. For the remainder of his life Pinel labored at the reorganization of the Salpêtrière, which he described as a 'picture of disorder and confusion.' By the time Charcot took command in 1862 in Pinel's original post of physician-in-chief, a long list of distinguished alienists had done valuable curative and research work, including Esquirol and Pariset. Among the physiologists occurs the great name of Magendie. As Charcot said in his 1867 lecture, the Salpêtrière had contributed notably to the vast mass of material collected by Cruveilhier for the *Atlas d' anatomie pathologique*— a landmark in the history of analytical medicine and diagnosis. But the hospital's day of glory was yet to come.

CHAPTER II

The   Founder   Of   Neurology

ONE OF the successors to Charcot's professorial chair, Georges Guillain, emphasizes in his book on Charcot's life and work that it was Charcot who first established neurology as an independent discipline in the Faculty of Medicine at Paris and hence in the world : 'It was the clinico-anatomic approach to the nervous system, designed and developed by Charcot that created the foundations of neurology.'[1] Charcot's genius and productivity were of crucial importance in the transformation of the neurological scene between 1850, when his neurological studies began, and 1893, the year he died. In mid-century, medical textbooks devoted only a few pages to such topics as vascular, infectious, or degenerative diseases of the brain; brain tumors (inaccurately classified); and spinal-cord pathology (vaguely described), together with quite inadequate accounts of epilepsy, chorea, and tetanus. But at the end of the century, 'the entire framework of modern neuropathology had been structured and carefully illustrated. The major categories of neurologic disease had been distinctly identified and exquisitely correlated with their anatomic and pathologic substrata.'[2]

If we think of Charcot today, it is usually in connection with Freud and Janet whose careers overlap in time those of Einstein and De Gaulle. But it best puts modern science into historical perspective and emphasizes the rapidity with which it has developed, if we recall that in the year of Charcot's birth a legitimist Bourbon king was still upon the throne of France. Jean-Martin Charcot was born in Paris on November 29, 1825. His father was a coach-builder working in partnership with his father-in-law, and the family seem to have been comfortably off in a

29

modest way. Jean-Martin was the second of four sons. The eldest continued in the family business, and the two youngest went into the army. Jean-Martin was taught at the Lycée Bonaparte, but he lived at home. The family resided in a lively part of Paris, near the present Grands Boulevards. Charcot has left no reminiscences of his boyhood. All that is known is that he was quiet and reserved, and that he liked to spend much time in reading and drawing—interests he maintained throughout his life.

In 1844 (by which time an Orleanist king reigned), Charcot entirely at his own wish started medical training and lived as a student in the Latin Quarter. His time was spent either in study or in sketching. He was particularly skilful at doing good-humored but incisive caricatures of his contemporaries or any colorful personality he encountered. These drawings are still to be seen in the Charcot Library at the Salpêtrière and include caricatures of his fellow professors and himself made at various times during his career. All his life Charcot was a fine observer and a superb draftsman, sketching places and people wherever he traveled and supplementing his clinical notes with drawings of patients and finely executed anatomical diagrams; he had the highly developed visual memory of the professional artist. Henri Meige associated Charcot's gift of caricature with his gift of diagnosis and pathological classification : 'At first glance he was able to recognize some oddity . . . but, aside from the comic, does not the physician's art have as one of its goals the discovery of physical anomalies and making them perceptible to others?'[3]

Charcot obtained his medical degree with ease and, following normal practice, he entered the status of Externat des Hôpitaux, a grade in which the student normally has to spend two years before being nominated—if he is lucky—to compete with others for selection as Internat des Hôpitaux, which is the essential first step on the ladder of a career in medical teaching and research. Though his brilliance attracted attention in his first year, Charcot had to wait the customary two years to be promoted to an internship at the Salpêtrière in 1848. (This was the year France again became temporarily a republic, the Citizen King being replaced by Citizen Bonaparte.) Included in the list of new interns were Potain ('Papa Potain') and Charcot's lifelong friend and collaborator, Edmé-Félix Alfred Vulpian.

To what extent Charcot went to the Salpêtrière by choice in the first place is uncertain. However, it was not long before his scientific curiosity was roused by the abundance of case material there and the multitude of problems, at that time quite unintelligible, presented by neuropathology. 'When he saw all the wilderness of paralyses, tremors, and spasms for which no name or proper understanding existed [in 1850], he would say, 'Faudrait y retourner et y rester' (One should return there and stay there).[4] This first impression determined the whole of Charcot's subsequent career. However, his apprentice work as an intern, though oriented to pathological anatomy, was not directed especially toward neurology, and his doctoral thesis (presented in 1852) concerned the problem of distinguishing between chronic rheumatism and gout. Indeed, Charcot was the first to establish this distinction. His results were greeted with great interest and identified him as a searching clinician.

Charcot's scientific thesis exemplified many features that were fundamental to his life's work. Diagnosis must be differential, and minutely variant forms of the same disease must be differentiated from one other and from other diseases superficially resembling them. Diagnosis must be supplemented by correlation of clinical signs, however minute, with their anatomical or physiological basis of expression. To get insight, therefore, observation must be thorough in each individual case. One must have numerous cases before attempting a generalization. Whenever possible, clinical observation ought to be supported by laboratory tests; for example, tests for uric acid in the body fluids in order to differentiate gout from the various forms of chronic arthritis. Finally autopsies are eminently desirable when the occasion presents itself, as they enable determination of the underlying anatomical causes or the effects of a disease. Sometimes the anatomical features discovered are closely related to the cause of the disease; in other cases, anatomical peculiarities are an expression of the condition and reveal the basis of some of the symptoms. Knowledge of this sort aids symptomatology and diagnostic differentiation. All this is now commonplace, but Charcot's thesis was a pioneering effort in the fine art of bringing a complete battery of research methods to bear on the task of diagnosis visualized as a search for enlightenment as to the cause and the origin of symptoms.

Charcot's thesis, soon to be recognized as a unique achievement, was easily defended in his doctoral examination. He was appointed to the grade of *Chéf de Clinique* in the department of Professor Rayer, a distinguished pathologist and personal physician to relatives of the new Emperor Napoleon III. All French universities and medical faculties are state governed and financed. The imperial connection was destined to benefit both Rayer and Charcot, and the advancement of analytical medicine. The 'little Napoleon,' though originally a demagogue, was a man of goodwill, a benevolent and enlightened despot with a real appreciation of science. By imperial decree he made Rayer Dean of the Faculty of Medicine and in 1862 asked the Faculty what new professorships they required. 'None,' was the reply, 'the curriculum is perfect.' But in the face of protests from the Faculty, the Emperor created new chairs in histology, the history of medicine, and comparative and experimental pathology, the latter chair being awarded to Rayer.[5]

From 1853 till 1855, Charcot worked as hospital physician on Rayer's staff and also, as was normal, set up in private practice. Through Rayer's good offices he became private physician to the brother of Fould, the banker (later minister of finance). This connection, together with Charcot's own transcendent abilities, launched that private practice which was to become so famous. But though happy enough with Rayer, whom he revered, Charcot still wanted above all to move to the Salpêtrière. This was achieved in 1856, when he became *Médecin des Hôpitaux de Paris*. Admission to this grade is open only to *Chéfs de Clinique* of two years' standing after a successful conclusion to the *concours*, a competitive examination. A successful candidate was nominated as one of the attending staff ('consultant physician' in English parlance) of one of the municipal hospitals. Such a post has no teaching duties, but is an indispensable step on the way to higher academic posts in the Faculty. French physicians of the rank of *Medicin des Hôpitaux* enjoyed, and usually availed themselves of, the privilege of transferring at regular intervals from hospital to hospital. Charcot never sought to leave the Salpêtrière and remained there six years as junior consultant.

During his first six years at the Salpêtrière, he produced a number of studies in general pathology reported in articles on

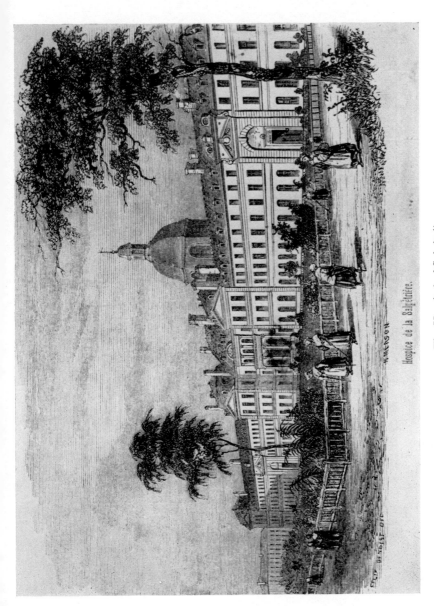

Hospice de la Salpêtrière.

The Hospital of Salpêtrière

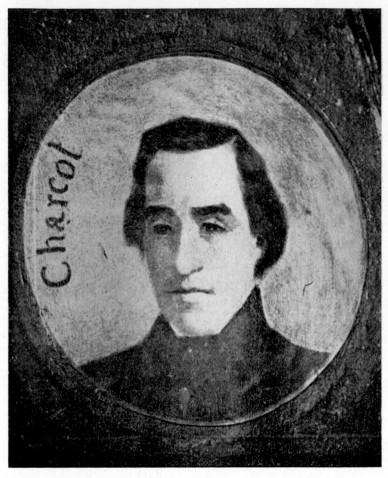

Charcot in 1848 when promoted Internat des Hôpitaux

typhoid, typhus and the plague as well as on diseases of the aorta and on chronic pneumonias. All this work was of excellent quality and thoroughness, but it gave no hint that later Charcot's attention would turn decisively to the pathology of the nervous system. This orientation became evident only in the years after his appointment as *Médecin de la Salpêtrière* in 1862. No longer in a subordinate post, as Chief of Medical Services in the hospital he occupied a position of freedom and authority. Now, at the age of thirty-seven, he had succeeded to the place once occupied by Pinel. He was free to reorganize much of the hospital for the benefit of both the inmates and medical research. Though not yet the holder of a teaching professorship in the University, his academic standing and prestige were reinforced by the title *Professeur Agrégé* won in 1860 in the severely competitive *Concours d'Agrégation*, in which he presented and defended a thesis entitled '*Intestinal Hemorrhages*.' He had failed in the *Concours* on a previous occasion, 1857, through nervousness during the oral presentation of a thesis significantly entitled '*The Expectations of Medicine*.'

On taking up his appointment as physician to the Salpêtrière, Charcot was delighted to find as his alternate and compeer his friend and contemporary, Vulpian, who had also been appointed a *Chef de Service*. In his *éloge* at Vulpian's funeral many years later, Charcot said : 'A perfect communion of feelings, ideas, and inclinations that even extended to the hardships of life, which were the same for both of us [in reference to their student and house-physician days] soon bound us together in a lifetime friendship.'[6] The two young savants made a survey of their vast and sprawling domain. The immense wards housed no less than five thousand displaced and crippled bodies and souls. Despite the concern of the great Pinel and two generations of his followers, improvement of conditions in the hospital had been slow. As late as 1838, the furious maniacs slept on the ground, and the helpless lay on straw, seldom attended. Rats still penetrated the low-lying cells and wounded the unhappy lunatics. Although these gross evils were gone by Charcot's day, grave problems remained. The world's greatest potential center for clinical neurological research was still merely a pandemonium of infirmities, a chaos of unclassified ailments, a mixed and mislabeled population. The patients fell into three broad categories (according to Charcot's description of 1867): First there were the mentally inadequate or disturbed comprising idiots, epileptics, and the insane. In addition there were 2,500 women who, 'for the most part, belong to the least favoured classes of society, but some of whom have known better days.' Some of these unfortunates were ladies of advancing age whom 'misfortune or desertion had placed under the protection of public charity,' but who enjoyed good health except in so far as the years were taking their toll. Charcot regarded these inmates as potential material for scientific geriatrics. The remainder of the patients comprised women of all ages 'affected for the most part with chronic maladies supposed to be incurable, and thus reduced to a state of lasting infirmity.'[7]

Charcot's aim was to identify each ailment as a clinical entity with a view to both understanding its etiology and taking appropriate measures of care and cure. Together with Vulpian, he commenced the heroic task of methodically examining every patient in every ward. The magnitude of that task explains some of the peculiarities of Charcot's method of working. He made his ward rounds with exemplary regularity, but he did not examine patients in the wards except when called to emergencies. Each morning for three hours he would examine patients in his office in the division of the Salpêtrière named after Pariset, the physician and man of letters who had been *Médecin de la Salpêtrière* until 1840. Professor Guillain describes Charcot's office as a small room, illuminated by a single window. The only furniture was a wardrobe for Charcot's hats, coats, and laboratory garb and a table and a few chairs. The walls were ornamented with some engravings by Raphael and Rubens and, in later years, with a signed portrait of the English neurologist Hughlings Jackson. The fact that the entire room and all its furnishings were painted in black tended, as Professor Guillain remarks, to produce a rather lugubrious effect. Be that as it may, Charcot's office certainly tends to vindicate Fred Hoyle's recent remark that great discoveries tend to be made in rabbit hutches rather than in glass palaces.

The patient would be brought to Charcot in his office. Sitting at his table, Charcot would listen attentively to a clinical summary of the case presented by an intern.

Then there was a long silence, during which Charcot looked, kept looking at the patient while tapping his hand on the table. His assistants, standing close together, waited anxiously for a word of enlightenment. Charcot continued to remain silent. After a while he would request the patient to make a movement; he would induce him to speak; he would ask that his reflexes be examined and that sensory responses be tested. And then again silence, the mysterious silence of Charcot. Finally he would call for a second patient, examine him like the first one, call for a third patient, and always without a word, silently make comparisons between them.

This type of meticulous clinical scrutiny, particularly of a visual type, was at the root of all Charcot's discoveries. The artist in him, who went hand in hand with the physician, played an interesting part in these discoveries.[6]

Pierre Marie, assistant in Charcot's private practice, who had also been in succession one of Charcot's interns and *Chéfs de Clinique* and ultimately followed Charcot in the Chair of Professor of the Diseases of the Nervous System, described Charcot as having a second sight so that he could almost sense or intuit a diagnosis. Even such a witness as Axel Munthe, who must be considered hostile and unfairly biased against Charcot, says that 'Charcot was almost uncanny in the way he went straight to the root of the evil, often apparently after a rapid glance at the patient from his cold eagle eyes.'[8] Munthe also says that apropos of his own promise as a clinician, '. . . even the Master with the head of a Caesar and the eye of an eagle mistook me for a rising man—the only error of diagnosis I ever knew Professor Charcot commit during years of watchful observation of his unerring judgement in the wards of his Salpêtrière or in his consulting-room in the Boulevard St Germain, thronged with patients from all the world.'[9]

Freud, who spent one year (1885-86) in study and observation at La Salpêtrière wrote interestingly on the subject in his obituary of Charcot in 1893.

He was not much given to cogitation, was not of the reflective

35

type [these slightly unexpected comments will merit discussion later], but he had an artistically gifted temperament—as he said himself, he was a *visuel*, a seer. He himself told us the following about his method of working : he was accustomed to look again and again at things that were incomprehensible to him, to deepen his impression of them day by day, until suddenly understanding of them dawned upon him. Before his mind's eye, order then came into the chaos apparently presented by the constant repetition of the same symptoms; the new clinical pictures which were characterized by the constant combination of certain syndromes took shape; the complete and extreme cases, the 'types', were then distinguishable with the aid of a specific kind of schematic arrangement, and with these as a starting-point the eye could follow down the long line of the less significant cases, the *'formes frustes'* [i.e., the appearance of the disease in patients where it was only partially manifested], showing some one or other peculiar feature of the type and fading into the indefinite.[10]

The problem of identification of the same basic disease occurring under variant manifestations in different patients was, and is, always an acute one. Biological material is essentially variable, and every individual reacts individually. Nowadays very sophisticated aids such as classificatory or discriminant analysis aided by computer programs are brought to the aid of the physician. Leaving aside the question of Charcot's supposed lack of reflectiveness, we can see from Freud's remarks that Charcot had the gift—which, clearly, he cultivated deliberately—of using his mind at the preconscious level as a 'computer' he could rely on if he gave it time and fed it with the requisite supply of comparative data. According to Freud, Charcot called this kind of mental work in which he had no equal *'practising nosography,'* work in which he took great pride.

He [Charcot] was heard to say that the greatest satisfaction man can experience is to see something new, that is, to recognize it as new, and he constantly returned with repeated observations to the subject of the difficulties and the value of such 'seeing.' He wondered how it happened that in the practice of medicine men could only see what they had already been taught to see; he described how wonderful it was suddenly to see new things—new diseases—though they were probably as old as the human race; he said that he often had to admit that he could now see many a thing which for thirty years in his wards he had ignored. No physician will need to be reminded of the wealth of new outlines which the science of neuropathology gained through his efforts, and of the much greater keenness and accuracy in diagnosis which was made possible by the aid of his observations. But to his pupils, who made the rounds with him through the wards of the Salpêtrière . . . he seemed a very Cuvier, as we see him in the statue in front of the Jardin des Plantes [the Paris Zoo, near the Salpêtrière], surrounded by the various types of animal life which he had understood and described.[11]

In his lecture of 1867, Charcot had mentioned nosography with reference to Pinel, who, he said, had been 'desirous of including Pathology [in medicine] in its whole extent and of creating a philosophical nosography, by applying to medicine the analytical method.' For both Charcot and Vulpian, the analytical method consisted not only in the careful visual observation of the patients, but in the study of what was happening in the *living tissues*. Strange as it may seem in those days it was exceptional for a hospital to have laboratory facilities, and there was not a single room in La Salpêtrière which was set aside as a laboratory. Charcot immediately remedied this deficiency. A room at the end of the cancer ward was set aside as a rudimentary research laboratory, furnished with a few microscopes. Before long it was cluttered up with glass jars reserved for the preservation of anatomical specimens. For a long time this was the totality of Charcot's meagre facilities, yet in a mere eight years he fashioned a magnificent series of masterpieces of research which established him by 1870 as the veritable creator of modern neurology.

Despite cramped working space and inadequate financing, Charcot eagerly brought in each new laboratory technique as it became known. It is difficult in the present century to realize just how new and rudimentary many processes such as photography were in 1860. The great atlases of anatomy such as Cruveilhier's consisted only of engravings in the early part of the century. Fortunately, Charcot was quick to appreciate the merits of a

37

free lance research worker—Duchenne de Boulogne. Duchenne had failed to obtain a Faculty appointment, but prior to 1862 did 'piecework' for several physicians including Broca and Rayer. This latter association put Duchenne into contact with Charcot, and in 1862 Charcot engaged him to work at the Salpêtrière in what was essentially a research capacity—a very unusual type of appointment in those days. There Duchenne learned microscopy and histology and in return yielded up all his secrets of medical photography. Since Duchenne was also a pioneer of electrophysiology, and interested in the electrical excitation of muscle, Charcot had valuable assistance in all matters of medical electricity in relation to diagnosis, research, and treatment. From 1870 onward, by which time Charcot had attained full recognition, his research facilities were constantly being added to. The original laboratory blossomed out into a cluster of research depots comprising a photographic studio, a workshop for making anatomic models, a histology center, a department for electrotherapy and electrodiagnosis, an eye and ear department, and a museum of pathological anatomy.

In Charcot's hands the clinico-anatomical method (as he called it) led to numerous fine and penetrating studies—the admiration of the time. Although the method had universal application, it could be employed with full force only in circumstances like those obtaining at the Salpêtrière; that is, in a hospital with numerous patients of all ages. Only abundant material can provide statistical facts reliable enough to provide a base for generalizations and inferences. If statistics are available, they often reveal facts to be quite at variance with views and presuppositions universally held and believed in. When Charcot and Vulpian first took stock of their patients they became interested in tremors, recognizing some of the instances to belong to Parkinson's disease (shaking palsy, paralysis agitans) but these symptoms did not especially relate to old age. When on another occasion Charcot decided that he wished to demonstrate senile tremors to his students, he searched the wards for examples but could find only a dozen cases. He therefore always maintained that, quite contrary to popular belief even among physicians, tremors are infrequent as the result of age alone. He would say,

Often playwrights depicted in their comedies old people as having excessive tremors of the head and of the limbs. This is a mistake that Shakespeare [Charcot's favorite poet whom he could and did quote extensively and appositely on the slightest provocation], a scrupulous observer in addition to being a great poet, knew how to avoid.[12]

Parkinson's disease was however the point of departure for a piece of research that was immediately acclaimed throughout the world. Charcot and Vulpian in the period of 1861-62 became aware of another disease that evoked tremors but was confusable with parkinsonism, and which he named 'multiple sclerosis.' The results were interesting from many points of view even to a non-clinician. Multiple sclerosis is, in fact, one of the commonest disorders of the nervous system. Prior to 1860, anatomists had recognized that some individuals have abnormal structures called 'pathologic plaques' in the nervous system, but no clinician prior to Charcot had been able to detect in the living human being a disease corresponding to their presence. It was left to Charcot to show that these plaques are in fact characteristic of multiple sclerosis. His was the first full description of parkinsonism as well as of the new disease, and he showed how differential diagnosis could be made. Several points of universal generality and of applicability to a wide range of human biological problems emerged. Each disease is a *syndrome* : that is, there are numerous effects on the patient which he can manifest in varying degrees. Thus the very tremor that was in the first instance definitive of Parkinson's disease can in undoubted sufferers from this ailment be so slight as to be practically nonexistent. Similarly, Charcot called attention to abortive forms of multiple sclerosis. ' Actually there is not a single element of the symptom complex [syndrome] in question that could not be lacking, and therefore in these cases the picture of multiple sclerosis is reduced simply to a contracture of the lower extremities. . . .'[13] At the same time Charcot predicted, rightly, that the incidence of the disease would tend to increase as diagnosis became more accurate and distinct from the favorite loose description of chronic myelitis.

Charcot was well aware that the incidence of diseases often tends (spuriously) to increase as diagnosis improves. An amusing example was provided by the ailments called tabetic arthropathies, which are lesions of the bones and joints found in locomotor ataxia (i.e., tabes dorsalis). After Charcot had drawn attention to these bone changes, English medical men gave the condition the name 'Charcot's joint,' Charcot having described it at a congress in London. (It was also called, 'Charcot's disease,' but this is best reserved for amyotrophic lateral sclerosis, a disease Charcot suddenly recognized as a new clinical entity in 1865.) His description, regarded as a masterpiece, has remained unmodified to the present day. Sir James Paget expressed his skepticism as to the existence of the arthropathies in a letter, presenting his doubts in veiled form, probably for politeness' sake. He asked if it was not a disease that was manifesting itself, if not for the first time, then with much greater frequency in the last few years than formerly. He based his inquiry on the rarity of bone specimens displaying these lesions in the British medical museums.

'Charcot's joint' won acceptance, but it is not surprising that pathologists of a later generation tended to reject as real clinical entities some of the diseases he defined. However, these rejections cannot be accepted uncritically. In 1876, Charcot described a 'new' disease under the name *tabes dorsal spasmodique*. It is a condition of slow onset, which develops between the ages of thirty to fifty, more commonly in men. A 'heaviness' of the legs is followed by a paresis accompanied with rigidity. Finally the gait assumes a spastic character and the patient becomes bedridden, but only after many years. Two reasons can be advanced with plausibility to explain skepticism as to the existence of this condition : First, Charcot remarked, unlike multiple sclerosis in which plaques are found in the nerve cells, and unlike many nervous diseases that are correlated with visible degeneration or abnormality of nervous tissue, *tabes dorsal spasmodique* provided no postmortem evidence of physical changes or pecularities. Second, no infective, metabolic, toxic, or vitamin deficiency etiology has been correlated with the condition. Many neurologists therefore tend to dismiss *tabes dorsal spasmodique* as a separate clinical identity, but ascribe the condition to either syphilitic myelitis or multiple sclerosis. Professor Guillain, however, believes that he has encountered patients presenting Charcot's clinical picture who, having been assayed by all modern clinical biological and serological examinations, represents neither cases of syphilitic lesion nor of multiple sclerosis.[14] Some other discoveries of Charcot's have been voted out of existence as a simple consequence of a change of name! For example, Charcot and Bouchard described cerebral lesions known as 'miliary aneurysms.' Although nowadays they are said to be rare or non-existent, Professor Guillain points out that they are now classified as 'vascular dilations.'[15]

As will be seen from the example of *tabes dorsal spasmodique*, numerous nervous, muscular, and bone diseases are of slow development, perhaps stretched out over decades, and showing great variability in the age of onset. To establish such maladies as clinical entities differentiated diagnostically from one another requires therefore not only large numbers of patients, but patients of all ages. As Charcot stressed in his 1867 course of lectures, at the Salpêtrière staff and students had the most favorable conditions for studying diseases of slow development; they could follow the unfolding of a disease through its entire course. What was also important was that in post-mortem examination they could detect the structural lesions at the root of the ailment. As the majority of chronic invalids who died in the Salpêtrière were without property or much encumbered by relatives, it was natural enough that their bodies should usually be available for the post-mortem examination to which Charcot attached such great scientific importance. This is the basis of Axel Munthe's nasty remark that Charcot was indifferent to the sufferings of his patients and took little interest in them from the day of establishing the diagnosis until the day of the autopsy.[16] When later we come to examine Munthe's trustworthiness as a witness, we shall not find it impressive. His remark is, in any event, patently at variance with Charcot's aim of following the course of a disease, and each patient must have been examined by him many times.

There is, in fact, abundant evidence of the tender and feeling aspect of Charcot's personality. In his 1867 lectures, he reported with sadness that it was rare to get cures in his patients either by spontaneous remission or by the intervention of art, and that it was correspondingly all the more important to learn as much as possible concerning effective palliatives and measures of alleviation. As a result, Charcot tended to be criticized for excessive eclecticism in applying a wide range of possibly curative or alle-viative treatments such as drugs, baths, massage, electricity, magnetism, fomentations and so forth. This criticism focused on the traditional character of most of these remedies, because it gave no guarantee that these measures would be scientifically directed at the real causes of a disorder and, therefore, made it unlikely that the treatment would be effective. Certainly, Charcot knew this. Yet his concern was precisely to withhold from the patient nothing that was harmless in itself while possibly doing some good. In addition, he was concerned to alleviate both physical and mental pain. Many of the treatments tended to give temporary relief to discomfort. It is also humane in itself to give the patient attention; an hour spent in a treatment in itself means something. It is an event in a dull and circumscribed life. It involves an excursion from the ward to another part of the hos-pital and the seeing of new faces and the meeting of new acquaintances with whom to exchange a word. Most important of all, the patient feels that his case is not being disregarded or neglected. In a word, treatment is tantamount to sympathy. Charcot, of course, looked for positive treatments of real value and pioneered the application of numerous drugs. He used silver nitrate for therapy in tabetic arthropathies and hyoscine to treat Parkinson's disease, a method still employed today. Indeed, he came under criticism from the opposite direction for being too keen on trying new procedures.[17]

The 'Caesar of the Salpêtrière' was in many ways exceptionally 'tender-minded' in the sense of William James's phrase, rather than 'tough.' His method, comparative and continued observ-ation followed by ultimate post-mortem, resulted from no ghoul-ish attitude toward the living or the dead, but was in correspond-ence with his attitude toward vivisection. His countryman Descartes, having reinforced the medieval doctrine that animals have no souls, had thereby encouraged animal experimentation to the grief of some of his contemporaries such as the humane Dr Henry More of Cambridge. Charcot respected Claude Bernard and Pasteur and saluted the experimental method, but he viewed major experiments on living animals with profound distaste. He loved animals passionately. According to Axel Munthe, 'He always cut short any conversation about sport and killing animals.' Munthe goes on to say: 'His dislike of the English derived . . . from his hatred of fox hunting.'[18] In truth, Charcot had no dislike for the countrymen of Shakespeare and William Harvey. He was always respectful toward English medicine past and present and had many English friends, such as Hack Tuke, nor did he judge men by their race or nationality. He well understood the ambivalence of the English among whom were at one and the same time the persecutors of foxes, hares, and stags; the opponents of vivisection; and the defenders of animals from cruelty. France, too, had its fox hunters at Fontainebleau and the chateaux of the Loire, equipped with huntsmen, horn, and redcoats. In the Second Empire, fox hunting was a recreation of the *haute bourgeoisie*. Also Charcot could not understand why his pupils Joffroy and Gombault liked to hunt, and he often reproached them for it publicly. The tracking down of an innocent creature to be chewed and torn to pieces by dogs was, said Charcot, a spectacle just as cruel as bullfights and just as anachronistic as the apparel of the hunters. Hunting of hares and foxes differed from bullfighting only in that the hunters did not run any risk.

Charcot was always careful not to agitate the minds of his patients by dropping casual words in the course of examination, or by showing too much outward interest in the pathology of a patient's condition. If necessary, he would speak in Latin. This caution was particularly important with sufferers from progressive diseases, because many of these conditions, though clinically detectable, develop so slowly as to be effectively benign, so that it would be an unnecessary piece of cruelty to upset the patients with information they would misunderstand in a pessimistic sense. Thus, in one of his Tuesday Lectures of 1887, Charcot said: 'I repeat there are forms of tabes that progress very slowly; I know people that have been tabetics for a long time but who are unaware of it. I shall not tell them: they will be unaware of their sickness, perhaps until their death.'[19]

It should be added that many benign forms of tabes and other diseases known to Charcot, when encountered again in the present century, have been claimed as new discoveries.

Charcot was always deeply disturbed when he came upon an acute disease that, being of a hereditary nature, was therefore likely to be incurable. Such a disease was peroneal muscular atrophy, discovered simultaneously by Tooth in London and Charcot and Marie in Paris. This disorder is an *abiotrophy* (a term coined by modern clinical geneticists), that is to say, a condition not congenital in the sense of being present at birth, but one coming on during life. The Charcot-Marie-Tooth disease usually begins in childhood, involving the feet and legs, and spreading some years later to the hands and the forearms. It is familial, being found in siblings, and is one of the first known examples of a heritable abiotrophy. In his lectures Charcot could never speak of acute incurable diseases without showing emotion. He would quote from the Greek tragedy,

What have we done, O Zeus! to deserve this destiny?
Our fathers were wanting, but we, what have we done?[20]

As a free thinker Charcot put forward no facile arguments to 'justify God's ways to man.' As a physician, he was extremely reluctant to record a fatal prognosis, even in patently hopeless cases.[21]

The savants at La Salpêtrière did not, of course, confine their attention to diseases of endogenous origin; they produced also many important findings in the field of toxic or infective conditions. Modern readers will be interested to know that the type of lesions involved in infantile paralysis, that is, poliomyelitis (then known as 'atrophic paralysis of childhood') were first located in Charcot's department. Duchenne, who had long studied the condition, in 1854 came to believe that the underlying lesions were located in the central nervous system. In a formidable piece of teamwork involving Vulpian, Prévost, and Corneil, Charcot and Joffroy finally showed that the principal symptoms of the disease (flaccid paralysis and muscular atrophy) result from atrophic lesions of the anterior horn cells of the spinal cord.

Detailed discussion of the vast subject of hysteria and related topics is reserved for a later study, but some points are worth noting in the present context. Hysteria is a protean entity manifesting the most diverse symptoms ranging from hallucinations through convulsions to paralyses, rigidities, and enervations. One of the special feats of Charcot's school was to show that hysteria-

44

like conditions occurred in men as well as women. Indeed, Charcot says that a surprisingly large number of men were admitted to the Salpêtrière.[22] It became necessary to discover whether the condition of these men was truly hysteria and thus presumably endogenous. A large proportion of these men were manual workers, and many of the conditions found in them were shown to be of toxic origin : either industrial poisoning as by lead, or excessive ingestion of alcohol. There remained, however, a residuum of cases not ascribable to exogenous effects which constituted the historic and definitive demonstration of the occurrence of hysteria in the male sex.

Charcot had a passion for teaching, and from the moment he became *Médecin* to the Salpêtrière he gave lecture courses in an improvised lecture room at the hospital. These courses were given without remuneration or special recognition. Attendance was optional and the audience, as were Charcot's own students at that time, was few in number. But, with each year that passed, the course became better known and attendance grew rapidly. Professor Vulpian became Professor of Pathological Anatomy in 1867. His rank was now that of Professeur de Chaire (full professor, i.e., a professor who is the head of a teaching department). Very few French teaching physicians ever reach this grade. In 1872, Vulpian was promoted to Professor of Experimental Pathology, and Charcot suceeeded him as Professor of Pathological Anatomy. Charcot's courses were well rounded and thorough and highly popular with the students, being masterpieces of clarity and thoroughness, and very carefully illustrated with anatomical specimens, diagrams and histological specimens. While much of his course had to do with routine knowledge to be communicated as effectively as possible to medical students and interns, Charcot also included much original matter of perfect freshness, reporting recent discoveries many of which were his own.

Professor Petulle, one of Charcot's successors in this Chair, wrote to Babinski in 1925 :

The audiences of Charcot still cherish today, after the passage of fifty years, the memory of his lectures which he gave with such clarity and performed with such persuasive authority, so that the

45

ideas of the master still remain dominant and permanently fixed in their minds. . . . He developed a true anatomicoclinical methodology. The impetus given by Charcot to the science of pathologic anatomy at the end of the nineteenth century was enormous.[23]

Charcot's concept of pathological anatomy regarded the subject as more than the servant of pathology alone. He had the creative vision to see that pathology holds a key to the understanding of the way in which the *normal* organ or organism functions. By study of the deranged, abnormal and malfunctioning organ we can learn something of how the normally functioning organ works. Thus Dr Rist, Secretary-General of the Paris Society of Hospital Physicians, was able to say at the 1925 Charcot Centenary Celebrations that Charcot

> . . . was one of the first to bring order to the immense collection of facts and documents that normal and pathological histology had accumulated. . . . And he was the first . . . to make . . . comprehensible syntheses of the intrinsic architecture of our organs as well as of their functions and of their diseases. The notions of the pulmonary lobule, the hepatic lobule, and the renal lobule were the fruits of this research which he undertook in order to create what he called 'the normal anatomy of structure.' How fertile these notions were. . . . One should, to keep them properly in mind, retrace the history of fifty years of medicine.[24]

Charcot occupied this Chair for ten years, until 1882. Meanwhile he continued his old informal lectures at the Salpêtrière. At the beginning of this period, although this set of lectures was well attended, Charcot still had relatively few clinical pupils at the hospital. Professor Debove, who spent a year as an intern with Charcot in 1873, found that the time passed for him almost entirely in intimate conversations with Charcot, which were always scientific, but not always exclusively medical. But in the next decade Charcot's teaching and research won international acclaim, and pupils flocked to the Salpêtrière from France and abroad, establishing the famous 'School of the Salpêtrière.' The roster of names of his pupils and junior collaborators reads like a list of authors of medical textbooks, for so many of these young men won fame either as partners of Charcot or later on their own. Yet, as Freud tells us: 'The "school of the Salpêtrière" was, of course, Charcot himself; his wealth of experience, his power of plastic description, his transparent clearness of diction was easily recognizable in the papers of every one of his pupils.' Freud also records an anecdote showing how Charcot's students were always reminded by him of the primacy of facts. One day a group of students brought up in the ways of German orthodox physiology grated on him by raising objections to his clinical observations. 'That cannot possibly be,' one of them interrupted, 'it contradicts the theory of Young-Helmholtz.' They were deeply impressed when Charcot replied simply 'La théorie, c'est bon, mais ça n'empêche pas d'exister."[25] ('Theory is fine but it doesn't stop things from existing').

In 1881, when Napoleon III had long come and gone, 'the circumstances of Charcot's life took on their final form. The idea came to be generally realized that the activity of this man was part of the national *gloire* to be guarded all the more jealously since the unsuccessful war of 1870-71.'[26] On a motion by Gambetta, the founder of the Third Republic, the Chamber of Deputies, of which he was president, voted the sum of 200,000 francs to establish a Chair of Diseases of the Nervous system. This was the first recognition anywhere in the world of neurology as an autonomous discipline. As intended, Charcot was appointed to the post in 1882. The Chair of Diseases of the Nervous System was to be held at the Salpêtrière, and a large amphitheatre was built there for Charcot's new official lectures. In addition, a general outpatient department was provided as well as a special inpatient division (devoted to nervous diseases only), with admission of both male and female patients. Charcot's official Medical Faculty Lectures were given on Fridays in the new lecture theatre. His old informal lectures, which had continued for twenty years in parallel with his course on pathological anatomy, delivered as *Professeur de Chaire*, were transferred to Tuesdays in the new outpatient department. These *Leçons du Mardi à la Salpêtrière* became as famous as the Friday ones. Both courses became the object of controversy and propaganda with

47

regard to the topics of hysteria and hypnotism. These subjects, of course, constituted only a fraction of the content of the lectures, and the record is very much distorted. It will, however, be advantageous to postpone objective discussion of these courses.

Charcot's actual research work had proceeded according to the sequence general pathology to neuropathology. He was not thought of as especially a neuropathologist until the late sixties of the century. But his original resolve as a student to return and stay at the Salpêtrière certainly did result in part from his interest in neurology. In fact, Freud reports that Charcot made his first observation in this field during his student days :

> Chance brought him into contact with a charwoman who suffered from a peculiar form of tremor and could not get work because of her awkwardness. Charcot recognized her condition to be 'choreiform paralysis,' already described by Duchenne, of the origin of which, however, nothing was known. In spite of her costing him a small fortune in broken plates and platters, Charcot kept her for years in his service and, when at last she died, could prove in the autopsy, that 'choreiform paralysis' was the clinical expression of multiple . . . sclerosis.[27]

Incidentally, one can hardly escape the conclusion that this act of Charcot's exemplified not only the single-mindedness of a scientist, but the deed of a kindly man.

As we have seen from his lectures on pathological anatomy, neuropathology led him on to general neurology. And in his last phase, study of the *neuroses* ('nervous' diseases unaccompanied by any discernable anomalies in the nervous system) led him beyond the structural and to the frontiers of psychology. When Freud calls Charcot 'unreflective,' Freud is perhaps being (unintentionally) misleading. Charcot was a great reader in many languages and, according to Léon Daudet, he was like Goethe or Montaigne—a man who radiated interest in everything. But there was a certain practical bias to his mind. He liked things hard and sharp, clear-cut and defined, not vague and formless. And possibly Freud only meant to say that Charcot was not given to philosophizing in the Germanic way—not even in the styles of Kant or Goethe. Charcot therefore would read philosophy of that kind which used to be called moral and ethical—human philosophy, 'humane studies' inclusive doubtless of the spirit of both David Hume and William James—but not metaphysics which to him seemed Hermetic.[28] He did not care to wander among concerns that were by definition obscure, or to voyage in a land of mist. To his logical Gallic mind it was pointless to ask Nature those questions to which she was deaf. Something of a French rationalist (in the nineteenth century sense of the term, not that of the Cartesian and Leibnizian philosophers), Charcot stopped on the hither side of transcendental speculation : The *Summa Theologica*, the *Principles of Philosophy, Transcendental Critiques* and the *Phenomenologies* of this, that and the other, doubtless seemed to him but as ropes of sand cast ineffectually toward the moon.

But philosophy, in its human aspects, and psychology were among Charcot's lifelong interests. A few months before his death in 1893, apropos of a discussion on psychological questions, he gave Janet a copy of Hartley's *Observations on Man*. The two volumes, full of psychological and moral discussions that even many philosophers had not read, had annotations from cover to cover. Janet being rather surprised at this, Charcot showed him a section of his library containing most of the contemporary books on psychology similarly annotated. In fact, Charcot was deeply concerned to develop a new approach to psychology. As he himself said, until the present (1885) physiologists had been in the habit of treating psychology lightly. Academic psychology was a small, superficial kind of psychology of no practical value. Another type of psychology ought to be created in correlation with pathophysiological studies. This could be attempted in cooperation with psychologists who themselves wished to break away from the introspective method of the past, in which the psychologist made himself the subject of his own investigation. In a more objective type of study, thought Charcot, the pathology of the nervous system would play an important role.[29] Thinking as he did, Charcot was willing to be made president in 1885 of the newly formed Society of Physiological Psychology, Jules, Janet, and Ribot being made vice-presidents. The secretary was Charles Richet, soon to become professor of physiology and in due course a Nobel Prize winner, as well as a writer on general subjects and a leading figure in psychical research. The Society had a broadly based membership comprising physicians, philosophers, writers and even poets. Too diversely composed to hold together for long unless centered in a figure as commanding as Charcot, the Society eventually disintegrated. However, it was in existence long enough to perform one notable service. It organized the first Congress of Psychology, which was held in Paris in 1889. The date was significant in that it came at the end of the decade that saw not only the rise of the physiological approach, but also the founding of the world's first laboratories for experimental psychology (by Wundt at Leipzig in 1879 and by Stanley Hall at Johns Hopkins in 1881) and the introduction of the experimental method at Harvard by William James.

Although Charcot encouraged as wide a circle as possible to take interest in physiological psychology and the general problem of the 'mind,' his own attack was directed at the role of the brain in various human faculties and capacities. In addition to the normal intake of interns engaged in the routine running of the hospital and who were being trained in neurology, Charcot encouraged collaborators with psychological interests to work at the Salpêtrière and employ its facilities for research. One of these protégés was Broca, one of the many brilliant men French science was producing at that time (from 1870 onward). Paul Broca was Professor of Surgical Pathology in the Faculty and later Professor of Clinical Surgery. Incidentally, having been a pupil of Lombroso's, he was the founder of physical anthropology in France, and originated scientific craniology. Broca maintained a continuing interest in the skull and its contents, a pursuit that brought him into frequent contact with Charcot at the Salpêtrière.

'Who?' said Charcot in his 1867 introductory lecture, quoting Hippocrates, 'could have foreseen from the structure of the brain that wine can derange its functions?'[30] Then he was speaking generally concerning empirical and causal medicine. But truly, to look at the brain, even when dissected into its parts, told one next to nothing of how it exercised its detailed functions. Charcot often looked at brains (indeed, there is an excellent cartoon showing him in apron and top hat with a brain in his hands, sketched in the autopsy room by Brissaud—then a mere extern who later became a professor on the Faculty), but he knew that the clinico-anatomic method was the only route to knowledge. The notion of localization of brain function had suffered by resemblance to the pseudoscience of phrenology. In the textbooks existing in 1860, the doctrine of Flourens (1794-1807) was accepted, and the brain was regarded as a homogeneous organ in which all parts were functionally equivalent. It was supposed that disturbances due to damage were proportional to the amount of tissue impaired. But a few researchers who had electrically stimulated the brains of experimental animals maintained that stimulation of different zones of the cerebral cortex produced different functional responses.

Charcot reinforced his instinctive detestation of vivisection with the pertinent remark that the brains of animals are not identical with those of humans. He was quite aware of Galen's mistakes based on dissection of the monkey. He was unimpressed by, and faintly sarcastic about, the 'decerebrate-cat' type of experiment. The 'school of the Salpêtrière' therefore applied to brain localization its typical method of making haste slowly by long-term study. Any symptoms of brain dysfunction exhibited by a patient were carefully recorded during life and eventually correlated with any brain lesions found at postmortem. Today we tend to couple the names of Lashley and Pinfield with brain localizations, but it should be realized Charcot's studies were of primary importance. Hardly a year went by without some new result being announced in this field, and Charcot's scientific communications on cerebral localizations were very numerous. Before summarizing Charcot's more notable results, it is worth mentioning the topic of aphasia.

Aphasia is sometimes congenital, but more frequently results from brain lesions or pressures due to brain tumors and is an inability to fully employ or understand language. It is a very variable condition. Whereas some aphasics can read or write words they cannot say, others can speak but not understand written words, or in other cases spoken words. In short, any combination of partial or complete loss of the skills of speaking, writing, reading, or understanding speech is a possibility. Charcot included some lectures on aphasia in his courses. In a lecture in

1883 he considered word-blindness (inability to recognize the written word) and on the basis of some clinico-anatomic observations he tentatively located it (i.e., the lesions for this dysfunction) in the inferior parietal lobules of the cortex with a possible extension to the angular gyrus and the first temporal convolution (i.e., the superior temporal gyrus). Charcot was very cautious in the matter of aphasia, and today his caution seems well justified, because it is admitted that while certain parts of the cerebral cortex are somewhat more critical for language skills than others, the localization is not very specific or very constant as among individuals. Disturbances in corresponding areas may produce different effects, and disturbances in different areas may produce similar effects.

Charcot had an instinct for being right and for avoiding leaps to unwarranted conclusions. He was therefore very reticent concerning Broca's theory that aphasia is localized in the (left) inferior gyrus of the frontal lobe. This doctrine was contested by Trousseau, one of the physicians in the Paris hospital service who had an aphasic patient. Adèle Anselin, as this patient was called became quite a medical celebrity in respect of her malady. When the day of her postmortem at length arrived the results were awaited with intense interest. This was so partly on account of Adèle's fame, but also because the autopsy was to be performed by Bouchard, who was destined to be a professor and, though only an intern at the Salpêtrière, was already a noted man locally. Numerous lesions were found in Adèle's brain, but the inferior frontal gyrus was quite intact. A further blow was delivered by Charcot in 1863, when he reported an autopsy performed by Corneil on an aphasic in the presence of Broca himself. Several gyruses were found to be degenerate, but the process had entirely avoided the inferior frontal one. Broca was stunned and, for a time at least, considered revising his theory. As for Charcot, Pierre Marie (his last Chief of Clinic), when asked about localization of aphasic disturbances, said merely that Charcot was not certain and hesitated to give an opinion.

Charcot concentrated on discovering the motor areas of the brain. He proved conclusively as early as 1875 that the brain is not homogeneous, but an association of functionally distinct parts. He was the first to locate the motor areas of the brain. In

1883 he and his pupil Pitres (later professor at Bordeaux) analyzed all available published data and demonstrated that the lower half of the precentral gyrus correlates with movements of the arm and face, while the upper half correlates with arm and leg. Some arm movements of restricted type are under the motor control of the middle frontal gyrus. Some movements of the face and motion of the tongue are referable to very restricted regions of the frontal area. Certain rather restrained areas of the paracentral lobule also control some leg movements. Charcot also realized the importance of Jacksonian epilepsy. In one of his *Leçons du Mardi* he pointed out that *partial* epilepsy (as it was called) had actually been discovered by Bravais at La Salpêtrière about 1828. However, Hughlings Jackson had studied this class of epilepsies in such a special way that he, Charcot, proposed to call it Jacksonian epilepsy. It has been so called ever since. A Jacksonian seizure is a spontaneous brain discharge that is confined to a restricted area of the cortex and therefore does not overwhelm the patient to the same degree as a major epileptic fit in which consciousness is lost. The patient in a Jacksonian seizure experiences sensory and psychic hallucinations and has only some of his motor functions disturbed, for example, a single limb may go out of control. Charcot apropos of Jacksonian epilepsy, anticipated the modern development of remedial neurosurgery and looked forward to the time when the kind of work which today we associate with the name of Pinfield would be, if not commonplace, well within the limits of surgical practice.

Charcot's studies on cerebral localization had effects of primary importance on the development of neurology and are among his greatest achievements. But it is difficult to single out any one of his many masterpieces as the crowning success in his life's work. As Freud said, there were few questions of any significance to which the School of the Salpêtrière had not made signal contributions. Like Augustus, who 'found Rome clay and left it marble,' the *Caesar de la Salpêtrière* had 'entered neurology in its infancy and left it at its coming-of-age, largely nourished by his own contributions.'

But his last decade saw yet other triumphs, unique among Charcot's researches in that their validity was disputed in his own time and after his death. But in reality Charcot's work on the neuroses was all of a piece with everything else he did—exact, incisive, and laying the foundation for a new science.

CHAPTER III

The Discovery of the Neuroses

IN THE second half of the nineteenth century the term *neurosis* came into use to denote any condition that apparently related in some way to the functioning of the nervous system but for which no organic basis had been discovered; that is no structural abnormality of the brain or nerves, nor any toxic or chemically determined state of the tissues. From the point of view of diagnosis or teaching, therefore, a neurosis tended in the minds of physicians or teachers of medicine to be an unsatisfactory entity, lacking clear-cut definition. For this and other reasons, neuroses were late of acceptance as fruitful objects of study in causal medicine. As Charcot said in his Inaugural Lecture when admitted to his new Chair of Diseases of the Nervous System in 1882 :

> Epilepsy, chorea, hysteria . . . come to us like so many Sphinxes
> . . . symptomatic combinations deprived of anatomical substratum do not present themselves to the mind of the physician with that appearance of solidity, of objectivity, of affections connected with an appreciable organic lesion.
>
> There are even some who see in some of these affections only an assemblage of odd incoherent phenomena innaccessible to analysis, and which had better, perhaps, be banished to the category of the unknown. It is hysteria which especially comes under this sort of proscription.[1]

Here Charcot adumbrates two mutually reinforcing reasons why the neuroses failed to attain full recognition and status as clinical entities. Each type of neurosis is highly variable in its expression. Neurasthenia, in combination with hypochondria, presents itself as the vaguest bundle of symptoms, and each neurasthenic comes to the physician with his own highly individual list of ailments. Axel Munthe, describing his patients at his practice in the Avenue de Villiers, says they would produce from their pockets little pieces of paper and read out an interminable list of symptoms and complaints—*le malade au petit papier*, as Charcot used to call it.[2] Sydenham in the seventeenth century characterized hysteria as 'the Proteus that cannot be laid hold of.' The protean nature of hysteria is exemplified by one of Mesmer's cures of an indisputable hysteric who suffered from convulsions, vomiting, diarrhea, urinary difficulties, toothache, and earache. However, the vagueness and variability of neurotic syndromes would not by themselves have been sufficient to relegate them to the back of the medical mind had an anatomical basis been discovered. If a histologically apparent abnormality such as the sclerotic plaques had been correlated with only a few cases of hysteria, for example, it would have created a profound impression, being a fact easy to reproduce in lectures and textbooks.

With some exceptions, therefore, the very existence of neuroses was hardly suspected outside the more sophisticated centers such as Paris and London. In the (medically speaking) provincial places, the differential diagnosis of one neurosis from another or between neuroses and disturbances with known organic bases remained a little known art. Freud said of himself in the period 1882-1885, when he was a junior hospital physician in Vienna :

> Fame of my diagnoses and their post-mortem confirmation brought an influx of American physicians. I understood nothing about the neuroses. On one occasion I introduced to my audience a neurotic suffering from a persistent headache as of chronic meningitis; they quite rightly rose in revolt against me, and my premature activities as a teacher came to an end. By way of excuse I may add that this happened at a time when greater authorities than myself in Vienna were in the habit of diagnosing neurasthenia as cerebral tumors.[3]

There was more than a little excuse for Freud and his masters, and Charcot himself explained the reason in his Inaugural Lecture. Neurotic symptoms, he said (and no one could say so with more authority than he), often matched to a high degree of resemblance those belonging to maladies having organic lesions. The similarity was at times so striking as to render differential diagnosis very difficult. He gave as examples the mimicry of a partial anesthesia of the skin by an anesthesia due to a brain lesion and some hysterical spasmodic paralyses that mimic those due to defects in the spinal cord. But, though an excuse in Charcot's eyes, this mimicry would be no justification for failing to aim at reliable differential diagnosis. He would not have approved of Meynert, Freud's professor at Vienna, who obstinately and quite fancifully classified mental diseases on a presumed anatomic basis and blamed melancholia and mania on disturbances either of cells of the cerebral cortex or of cortical circulation of the blood. Meynert represented the school of thought lasting to the end of the nineteenth century which has been appropriately called 'brain mythology.'[4]

Charcot's work on the neuroses was precipitated by an event in the domestic economy of the Salpêtrière which occurred about 1870. The buildings of La Salpêtrière had been perpetually added to since the time of Louis XIII, but none had ever been pulled down before it fell down. At last the Bâtiment Saint Laurent became so delapidated that evacuation became mandatory. In this building, which had belonged to the psychiatric service of Dr Delasiauve, epileptics, neurotics, and the insane had been housed together, pell-mell fashion. In the transfer it was thought wise to separate the insane (i.e., psychotics suffering from mania, melancholia, or schizophrenia) from the nonpsychotic epileptics and the 'hysterics.' The latter two groups, whose behavior (being episodic) had similarities, were housed in a new Quarter for Pure Epileptics, and Charcot as senior physician took the new service under his wing.[5]

The patients in the new 'epileptic ward' fell into three classes. One group consisted of true epileptics, who had seizures of such frequency and acuteness as to necessitate their permanent hospitalization. Another group consisted of nonepileptic severe neurotics classed under the blanket term 'hysterics.' A third group were epileptics who also were hysterical. The hysterics comprised

57

sufferers from a variety of syndromes that today would be sub-classified, the term 'hysteria' being a broad one. Patients with anxiety, phobias, or obsessive-compulsive neuroses were doubtless absent, though possibly represented in the outpatient department, when it was opened. The hysterical inpatients would have fallen into three classes : (a) sufferers from 'dissociative reaction' —somnambulism, fugue, ambulatory automatism; (b) victims of 'conversion reaction,' with a variety of physical symptoms or failure of function; (c) a proportion of patients with psychosomatic ailments, for example, endocrine-sympathetic disorders that today would not be classified as conversion hysterias proper.

In addition to these three groups, there might well have been a small proportion of schizophrenics and some sufferers from Kahlbaum's catatonia, which in part resembles *grande hystérie*. However, there is no reason to suppose that Charcot's service had any excessive tendency to diagnose hysteria. Dr Georges Guinon, analyzing the patients examined during one year, found that hysteria was diagnosed 244 times in 3,168 consultations. Professor Guillain remarks that, at his own consultations at the Salpêtrière in the present century, he made diagnosis of hysteria in exactly the same proportion as Charcot, with one difference only—the name : Modern practice is to call the condition *psychoneurosis* or *functional disturbance*. The patients have not changed since Charcot's time, only the terminology.[6]

Charcot himself tended as the years went by more and more to dislike the term 'hysteria' and to speak instead of 'neurosis.' The name 'hysteria' has a long history. In ordinary parlance, we think of hysteria as either a state of overanxiety or an attack of 'the hysterics'—excitable laughing or crying. The ancients regarded the condition as characterized by these latter attacks, which have, of course, from time immemorial occurred also in more violent and convulsive forms. Hysteria was regarded as primarily a female disorder, and the famous theory ascribed to Hippocrates referred its origin to *hysteria* (the uterus). Aretaeus, who lived in the first century AD, was more specific in asserting that the uterus is liable to be suddenly carried upward within the abdominal cavity. Violently compressing the vital organs, it gives rise to 'hysterical suffocation'—a choking sensation leading to a fainting fit. As will be seen, Aretaeus was familiar with at least one type of hysterical attack and described the premonitory signs or *aura* involving agitation, breathlessness, and *globus hystericus*. The idea of uterine migration was rejected by Galen, who substituted a theory of 'local suffocation' due to swelling of the uterus. But most of the medievals reverted to the notion of a wandering uterus and sought to lay it to rest by invocation or exorcism. Charles Lepois (1563-1633) insisted that the cause of hysteria is to be found in the brain, and that therefore men as well as women are liable to be subject to it. But twenty years later Lazare Rivière was still able to write a chapter 'De furore uteris' in his *Praxis Medica*, and until 1900 or so one could still find learned savants who were convinced that hysteria was a kind of uterine fury and an exclusively feminine weakness.[7]

It is likely that the medieval notion of the daughters of Eve as given to weak-minded fancies and as deceivers of honest Adams, which lingered on through Victorian times into the era of the suffragette movement, also played a part in the neglect of hysteria as an objective and serious ailment. There are two common views of neurosis : as self-deception, and as deception of others—malingering or 'putting it on.' Even in this day and age, we are familiar with the attitude that it is all the fault of the nervous or emotional sufferer for not 'exercising self-control,' not 'pulling himself together,' or 'letting herself give way to it.' Similarly, the view still persists that the neurotic is inventing his symptoms so as to get his way with his family, or is malingering to get industrial compensation or to delay a return to work. Of course, sometimes there is a grain of truth in these beliefs, but the matter is profoundly complicated in ways almost unsuspected a century ago, when the attitudes mentioned were prevalent among medical men as well as lay people. The pendulum had swung violently from the view that disorders were the work of demons to the opposite extreme, which tended to deny reality to at least the milder neuroses.

Janet characterizes the history of the study of hysteria as comprising three periods. Superstition, ignorance, and error gave way late in the nineteenth century to the clinical period, which at the close of the century yielded to the psychological period.[8] In the clinical period, 'physicians sought, above all, to give a medical character to this disease, to distinguish it from other maladies, and to recognize the phenomena that appertain to it. It is a kind of clearing away and classification.' When the opportunity to observe hysteria came his way, Charcot was of all persons the one specially qualified to classify, distinguish, and diagnose by virtue of two decades of work already oriented toward this end in organic neuropathology. Every life science, before it can attain maturity, must pass through the stage of accurate description and classification coupled with a search for correlations; that is to say, the discovery of laws. Hippocrates, in *The Sacred Disease* remarked :

Another strong proof that this disease [epilepsy] is no more divine than any other is that it affects the naturally phlegmatic, but does not attack the bilious. Yet if it were more divine than others, this disease ought to have attacked all equally, without making any difference between bilious and phlegmatic.

Whether the correlations perceived by the Hippocratics were true or not is of no concern. The point was simply that any correlations that exist demonstrate that a phenomenon has its laws and therefore belongs not to the sphere of the capricious, the irrational, or the supernatural but to the domain of the natural and is a proper object of scientific study.

When the hysterics at the Salpêtrière came under *Le service de M. Charcot*, the way to reliable knowledge of hysteria had been prepared by various clinical researches of high quality. The English physician Brodie, of whom Charcot thought very highly, had produced a beautiful book (as Janet called it) in 1837, drawing attention to the provenance of hysterical pains in women, hysterical stiffness of the knees ('Brodie's knee') and the fact that hysterical local conditions can ensue after very minor injuries. In France studies had been published by Brachet and Landouzy in 1845, by du Saulle in 1860, and by Charcot's own Duchenne de Boulogne in 1855. But the first general work of real value and the point of departure for the researches of the Salpêtrière was the *Traité clinique et thérapeutique de l'hystérie* published in 1859 by Pierre Briquet (1796-1881), a teacher in the Paris Faculty somewhat senior in years to Charcot and physician at La

Charité since 1846. In his Inaugural Lecture of 1882, Charcot said of hysteria, the Proteus :

> But we ought . . . to make the best of things as we find them, and not allow ourselves to be disheartened by the difficulties they present. A more attentive study makes us see things under an altogether different aspect.
>
> Briquet . . . established beyond dispute, that hysteria is governed in the same way as other morbid conditions by *rules* and *laws*, which attentive and sufficiently numerous observations always permit us to establish.[9]

Between his Inaugural lecture and his death in 1893, eleven years remained to Charcot. His official lectures from the Chair of Nervous Diseases occupy three volumes. It is interesting to see the amount of teaching he alloted to hysteria. Somewhat more than one-third of his lectures were devoted to hysterias and their comparison with (or contrast to) organically determined neuropathies. Charcot's interest extended much beyond the theoretical, for he took his responsibilities as a teacher seriously. He knew that what he had to say would be of the greatest practical importance to the future patients of his students, who were the future hospital physicians and general practitioners of Paris. In teaching in the Faculty of Paris, Charcot was, of course, teaching France and the world. He was concerned that the hysteric should receive the therapeutic treatment he deserved and be protected from treatment he did not need or deserve, such as the surgeon's knife—always apt in those days to leap from its scabbard. He was concerned that the genuine traumatic neurotic should get his sick pay and industrial compensation and not be rejected as a malingerer.

Charcot regarded his first duty as a teacher as acquainting the medical public with all the diverse forms of hysteria, including its more muted symptoms and obscurer signs. He was anxious primarily for objectivity. This for him was necessarily to be founded on the careful description of physical conditions, altered physiological and sensory capacities rather than behavioral signs. Both Charcot's passion for objectivity and his disinclination to run before he could walk have been somewhat misrepresented and exaggerated by numerous historians of medical psychology. The statement in one form or another has often been made to the effect that,

> Charcot 'thought only in terms of the nervous system. . . . Moreover, bent on being extremely scientific – which consciously or unconsciously still meant to base everything only on the functions of the brain and nerves – Charcot felt that the possibility of simulation would be thoroughly eliminated if the neurological signs of paralyses and anesthesias were carefully checked. . . . Freud, facetiously to be sure, adopted the jargon of Charcot's circle, the jargon which reflected the one-sidedness and prejudices which reigned in the minds of that active and industrious scientific group.'[10]

Even Freud is slightly misleading when he says of Charcot, 'It was easy to see that in reality he took no special interest in penetrating more deeply into the psychology of the neuroses. When all is said and done, it was from pathological anatomy that his work had started.'[11] Elsewhere Freud says much that corrects the impression that Charcot in his long study of hysteria thought only of nerve fibers and their connections.[12] But if one follows through Charcot's lectures in their entire course, one sees how—to a surprising degree—his views widened and broadened to the point where he spoke more and more in terms of 'functional' or 'dynamic' causes and explicitly of 'psychic' causes (i.e., psychological ones), so that in retrospect Janet could say that Charcot asserted that hysteria had a psychic origin. What is surprising in Charcot's development is not his devotion to the organic and the material, but his emancipation therefrom—an orientation that more than the contributions of any other school opened the door to the era of psychological interpretation of the neuroses.

But this conceptual change occurred at the end of the journey, not at the beginning. First came the objective description of the manifestations of the disorder. The diversity of expression can best be paraded before the reader by using Charcot's own summary given by him and Pierre Marie in the article 'Hysteria' written for the *Dictionary of Psychological Medicine* published in London in 1892 and edited by Charcot's friend, Hack Tuke, a physician who worthily upheld the Tuke family's concern for proper treatment of mental disorders. Charcot always had the liveliest regard and respect for Hack Tuke, and their relations were most cordial. The article is interesting. Written only a year before Charcot's death, it is concerned primarily with the problem of precise description, but in certain passages it comes extremely close to a predominantly psychological view of the *grande néurose*. In the article's introductory paragraphs there occurs early a strikingly modern sentence. 'What then is hysteria, . . . less a disease than a peculiarly constituted mode of feeling and reaction.' But he abstains from any psychological theory. He says merely, 'We do not know anything about its nature, nor about any lesions producing it.' It is noteworthy that he does not say *the* lesions producing it. He proceeds to describe the two broad forms of manifestation, the convulsive and the non-convulsive.

Convulsive attacks vary among patients and even within the same individual. But such variation occurs in most diseases and is not peculiar to neuroses. According to Charcot, a typical convulsive attack passed through three distinct stages : First came the *epileptoid stage*, which rarely came on entirely without warning, but was heralded by certain prodromata or premonitory signs. Sometimes there would be mental excitement and agitation and possibly hallucination, or a nervous cough, yawning, or tremor. But the most usual 'premonitory aura' consisted of palpitation with a sense of tightness in the head, a feeling of excessive warmth, and the famous 'globus hystericus'—a sensation of obstruction in the throat as of a ball rising there. A fairly common sign was the 'ovarian aura,' a sharp pain in the ovarian or some other region of the trunk. The epileptoid stage, usually of a few minutes' duration, commenced with the patient falling backward with loss of consciousness, weak breathing, swelling of the neck, and foaming at the mouth. Then came a 'tonic phase,' with the arms and legs stretched out and going into short and violent oscillations. This was succeeded by the phase of 'muscular relaxation,' in which activity subsided while full respiration was resumed. While these subsidiary phases could often be distinguished, they showed considerable variation in duration and intensity.

The supine patient next entered the second stage of disordered movements, sometimes called the *stage of clownism*. Often the body is bent in the form known as *l'arc de cercle*, analogous to that seen in tetanus, resting only on head and heels. Sometimes this posture passed over into that known as the 'salutation,' in which the patient repeatedly passes from the lying to the sitting position. Other gymnastics also took place often, says Charcot, quite surprising to watch in weak and unathletic patients.

In the quotation that follows, Charcot describes the third stage, which he named *attitudes passionelles*, as quite different from the preceding one and showing the 'psychical element,'

> The patient begins to give himself to expressive mimicry, indicating the sentiments . . . which move him; pleasure, pain, fear, even fright, love, hatred, etc.; not unfrequently this sentiment and mimicry are in relation to a vivid impression or an emotion formerly experienced by the patient, which often has played a part in the explosion of hysterical symptoms. In such cases we sometimes see the patient recall a whole scene in his former life (some dispute, accident, etc.). Mimicry mostly takes the first place, but some patients also scream in connection with their sentiments, and some make long speeches. The duration of this period is still more variable than that of the preceding ones.[13]

After the *attitudes passionelles*, the attack usually terminated or repeated itself, starting all over again in epileptoid form.

In some rare cases, a fourth stage occurred—that of *post-hysterical derangement* lasting a few hours or even days. The patient lay in a state of mental confusion and delirium, his thoughts moving in the same circle of ideas as those manifested in the *attitudes passionelle*.

At the Salpêtrière they found that in numerous patients the *grande hystérie*, as the convulsive attack was called, did not run through its full cycle. Any of the stages could be absent or occur merely in a muted form. In many patients also only a very few of the features of the *grande attaque* would manifest themselves: a few contractions of the hands and arms or legs; jerky breathing; and cries, tears, and sighs. Charcot and his colleagues called

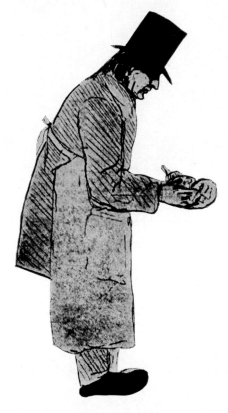

Charcot examining a brain. From a 1875 sketch by Brissaud

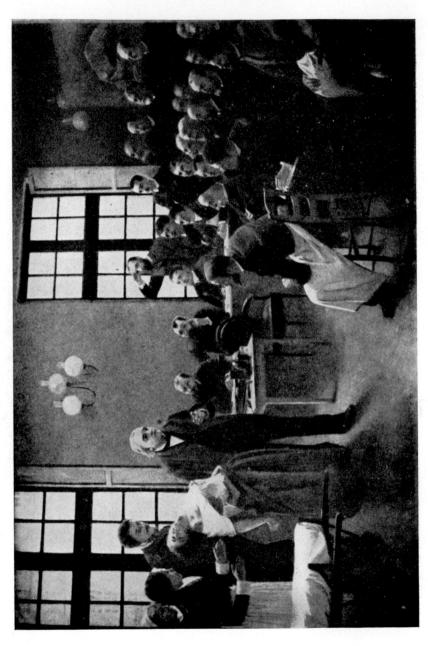

Demonstrating hysteria

these lesser attacks *hysteria minor* as opposed to *hysteria major*, the grand attack. But they insisted that there was no real difference of kind between major and minor attacks and that all transitional stages were to be found in the hospital wards.

In the twentieth century, the grand attack or *hysteria major* seems to have been observed in its entirety with decreasing frequency. In 1906 Janet was able to say that 'nobody nowadays any longer describes the attack of hysteria as Charcot did.' Janet hints at one possible reason when he says, 'No doubt, our types of hysterical phenomena are ephemeral like his.'[14] That is to say, its etiology being in the main psychological, hysteria is a socially malleable disorder, and the form and intensity of its manifestation tend to alter as the milieu changes. Other writers suggest that among the Salpêtrière patients were some catatonic schizophrenics whose catatonias might in some degree have resembled hysterical fits, especially the stage of clownism; they could well have been hysterical also. As remarked by Jung many years ago, there are difficulties in the differential diagnosis of hysteria and some schizophrenias. Indeed, some modern critics of psychoanalysis suggest that the discipline was founded on Freud's analysis of half a dozen patients who were not hysterical but schizophrenic.

But the schizophrenia hypothesis is not essential to explain why at least some of the patients in the epilepsy-hysteria wards should have had attacks comprising all three stages and perhaps even the fourth. Many of the patients were cases of long standing in which the disorder, by modern standards almost untreated, had become entrenched. In later years hysteria came to be diagnosed early and nipped in the bud by prompt treatment. This alone would greatly reduce the frequency of the grand attack. Hysteria thrived also in the wards of the Salpêtrière by suggestion and unconscious imitation—imitation not only of hysteria but of epileptic seizures. Charcot was quite aware of this phenomenon. He believed almost passionately in the value of isolation in the treatment of hysteria and deplored the limited resources that necessitated keeping hysterics together and in propinquity to epileptics. As time went on more segregation was achieved but it depended like all large scale medical improvements on the supply of money. In France funds came mostly from the state, which contributed increasingly out of the prosperity of the Third Republic. But, as in all places and times, the funds though welcome never came fast enough to please Charcot and his colleagues.

As Janet and others have said, Charcot's description of the *grande attaque* is possibly somewhat artificial in the sense that both the number of stages represented in actual attacks and, their order of occurrence were, in fact highly variable. Janet is right, however, when he approves Charcot's *'schéma'* as having been, at least momentarily, intelligible and useful. It fixed ideas and provided a point of reference, and as such 'did service to many a generation of students. It brought about an enormous scientific movement. . . .'[15] Although the grand attack in its programmatic unfolding is rarely seen, at least today, each sub-stage exists and is encountered in reality in some hysteric patient. This is true of the Hysteric Aura and of Globus Hystericus, of the fainting fit, of the convulsive limb movements, and of the *attitudes passionelles*. It is also true of the patient's amnesia concerning the events, that is the somnambulism or automatism of the seizure. Janet probably summed up the question fairly when he said in his lectures 'The Mental State of Hystericals' that the *grande attaque* occurred when the patient had several kinds of attack in short succession.

In his *Dictionary* article 'Hysteria,' Charcot goes on to emphasize that hysteria is by no means fully represented by the grand attack or even by the *formes frustes* (isolated episodes of convulsions or fits). There are somnambulisms in which the patient lives in a delirium, and ambulatory automatisms or amnestic fugues in which, although the patient's aspect and behavior are almost normal he seems to have no recollection of his ordinary identity and aims in life and loses recollection of what he has done in the fugue state as soon as he emerges from it. But these somnambulisms and fugues are clearly of a character similar to the stage of the *attitudes passionelles* in hysteria major, which has much in common with delirium and somnambulism as commonly understood. Charcot put great stress on the class of symptoms now called 'conversion hysteria.' In Charcot's experience, derangements of the sensory perceptions were among the most constant signs of hysteria. 'Anesthesias' involved

66

a lack of ordinary sensation in the skin and subcutaneous layers. Sometimes the whole body surface became insensitive to pain, heat, or electric shock. In other patients there would be hemi-anesthesia, the whole of one side of the integument being insensitive. In yet other cases a hand, an arm, or even a whole limb would lack superficial sensitivity. Special senses such as taste, smell, and hearing could be lost or diminished. Hysterical blindness was rare, but it was common for the field of vision to be contracted. 'Achromatopsia' was often found, the patient in extreme cases seeing all colors as tones of gray and in other cases being defective for some regions of the spectrum only.

'Algias' ('hysterical pains') such as Cephalgia (in the head), Gasteralgia (in the abdomen), Ovaralgia (in the ovarian region) and Arthralgia (in the joints) were innumerable.

Charcot lists various behavioral reflexes such as dry cough, sneezing, yawning, and hiccoughing. These are mild instances of 'Tics' (in a manner of speaking) and hence a motor phenomenon. They are analogous to muscular 'Spasms' such as the pulling aside of the tongue. Muscular 'Tremor' was frequent in hysterics, especially in or near a limb affected with hysterical paralyses or contractures. 'Hysterical Chorea' had been long recognized and consisted of rhythmic stereotyped movements. Hysterical 'Contractures' were numerous. A hand might be permanently bent at the knuckles or at the wrist, or a forearm permanently elevated, or a knee drawn up, or one leg crossed over the other.

'Flaccid Paralyses' were the reverse of spasms or contractures and most striking. Said Charcot:

> In the different forms of flaccid paralysis, the limb presents quite a different aspect, the arm hangs down motionless, its position being determined by gravity; it seems as if the head was drawn down by a heavy weight, whilst at the same time the shoulder is flattened. Spontaneous movement no longer exists, and the arm is like a foreign body over which the will has no influence, and if lifted it falls down at once. In the case of *crural monoplegia* the patient lies on his bed unable to make any movement with the affected leg; walking without support is impossible,

and if the patient walks on crutches the leg hangs down without motion, and is dragged along behind; it follows, so to say, the pelvis to which it is attached and scrapes over the ground.[16]

The strangest paralyses of all, more extravagant and unintelligible than the others, were constituted by 'Astasia,' the inability to stand upright, with 'Abasia,' the inability to walk. As a rule the subjects were young people with undiminished muscular strength and all the normal reflexes. When examined in bed they could execute all normal movements with normal strength, and it seemed there was nothing at all the matter with them. But they were absolutely incapable of walking, for if made to stand they would bend, twist their legs, and fall. 'In a few cases described by Charcot, the comedy is still more complete; they are able to make certain leg movements which seem very complicated—jumping, dancing, hopping on one leg, running—but they fall as soon as they try to walk.'[17] Other paralyses fall into the same type; a needlewoman can no longer sew, a pianist can no longer play the piano, even though there is no paralysis of the hand. It seems such patients have 'forgotten' a capability. As Charcot said of astasia-abasia, 'the patient has unlearned to walk.'[18]

Charcot as a 'visual type' attached great importance to accurate visual recognition of the form of neurotic symptoms and the signs of organic neuropathies. His lectures were profusely supplemented with every kind of illustration, diagram, photograph, and model. Charcot's son, Commander Jean Charcot, the explorer, describes Paul Richer as a devoted and indispensable collaborator of his father's. Richer was originally one of Charcot's interns, and from 1882 to 1895 he was chief of the Laboratory at the Salpêtrière. A distinguished artist, he made all the drawings and models for Charcot's lectures. Eventually Richer was appointed Professor of Creative Anatomy at the National School of Fine Arts (Ecole des Beaux Arts) while a member of the Academy of Medicine—a pleasing reflection on the meeting of cultures in the scientific metropolis of the world which was also the city of Rodin and Manet. In the period 1876-1880, Charcot had also seen into production, with a preface by himself, a work in several volumes by Bourneville and Paul

Régnard : *La Grande Hystérie; Iconographie Photographique de la Salpêtrière*, which was described by Castiglioni as magnificent, a classic in the eloquence of its style, in its clarity, and in the value of its contents.[19]

As a man of broad culture who felt the need to propagandize the objective reality of hysteria as a relatively constant phenomenon occurring in both sexes, Charcot collected historical material both in literary form and as visual representations of sufferers with hysterical or neuropathic abnormalities. In collaboration with Paul Richer he engendered a remarkable book, *Les Démoniaques dans l'Art*. In presenting this study before the Academy of Medicine in 1887, Charcot spoke of his objective in noting all the works of art—paintings, mosaics, tapestries, sculptures, icons, and bas-reliefs—which depicted anything to do with epileptics, ecstatics, choreics, possessed, and demoniacs. 'This retrospective study,' as he called it, 'demonstrated that hysteria is in no way, as some claim, a sickness typical of our century and that in the archives of the past there is also proof that it attacks the male as well as the female.' The Demoniacs was supplemented in 1887 by a further volume, *Les Difformes et les Malades dans l'Art*. Zilboorg claims that these studies were a great step forward in the history of medical psychology. Not only did they indicate the value of the historical-comparative method, but they showed that psychopathology might gain insight from the study of artistic self-expression. As the nineteenth century grew into the twentieth, this broadening of vision, whose initial impetus had come from Charcot, expanded into anthropology, sociology and literature.[20] In this connection we have only to think of the literary-historical-sociological essays of Freud and Jung.

In his writings and lectures, Charcot drew comparisons between contemporary cases of hysteria and some of the enigmas of the past. He attributed the great saltatory epidemics of the Middle Ages such as the dancing epidemics of Saint Guy and the *chorea germanorum* to Hysterical Chorea.[21] The ecstasies and so-called demonic possessions of former periods always interested him. He would always comment if he had a patient from some provincial place such as Louviers or Loudun which had been the scene of 'diabolical' transactions. Many of the suspected witches had anesthetic points, so beloved of such old witch-finders and witch-prickers as the English Matthew Hopkins, and Charcot equated these with the anesthetic areas found in so many hysterics, the lack of sensibility extending to some depth below the skin.

Charcot found dramatic earlier manifestations of hysteria in the convulsionnaires who had disported themselves almost on his own doorstep, namely in the churchyard of Saint Médard in Paris in the years 1727-1732. These strange people foregathered at the tomb of the Deacon François de Pâris, a Jansenist of great piety who died in 1727 at the age of thirty-seven from self-imposed starvation. This itself may have involved an element of hysteria, as hysterical anorexia (unwillingness or inability to eat) is rightly suspected of playing some role in the feats of some of the heroes of prolonged fasting. Be that as it may, the worthy Deacon was unlikely to attain to official sainthood, being tainted with heresy. Many of the Jansenist theological propositions (derived from the Dutch reformer Jansen, 1585-1638) had long been declared erroneous by the Vatican, but Paris still had a strong Jansenist movement. In 1713, the Pope delivered a further condemnation, but it was not until 1730 that the Parliament of Paris got around to registering it, thereby intensifying religious enthusiasm among the Jansenists. Since the death of the good Deacon, the sick and the poor had repaired to his tomb in the hope of cures and miracles, but from 1730 to 1732 the scenes in the cemetery were especially extravagant : people fell on the ground or leapt into the air in states of ecstasy; women twisted themselves into bizarre contortions. Eventually in 1732, Louis XV, fearing for public order, closed the churchyard and incarcerated the convulsionnaires in the prison of La Force at the Salpêtrière.[22]

When demonstrating Ovaralgia (pain in the abdomen, often in the ovarian region) Charcot spoke of the peculiar kind of treatment or *secours* meted out to convulsionnaires at Saint Médard 'at their own request.' This 'succour' consisted in the application of heavy blows on the abdomen delivered with heavy and fearsome instruments, or in intense pressure administered by either doubled fists, tight swaddling, or (most extreme of all) men sitting on the patient. Charcot commended Hecquet, a contemporary physician, who in the treatise *Du naturalisme des convulsions* discussed these remarkable happenings as being purely natural ones. Charcot had found that in some hysterics ovaralgia, no matter how intense and distressing, could be dramatically relieved by a firm but rather hard pressure or a fairly weighty blow. But his ovariform hysterias also tended to be characterized by anesthesia accompanied by a tendency not to bleed from minor injury to the skin. This explained the insensitivity of the succored convulsionnaires and also the odd fact that they did not bleed when given sword blows at their own request. This last could be quite true, said Charcot, if the edge did not penetrate too deeply.[23]

As a result of Charcot's historical comparisons, there grew up around him and La Salpêtrière a group of medical historians who interested themselves in the various manifestations of neurosis as diagnosed retrospectively from the *descriptions naïves* given in the literature of the marvelous. Among Charcot's friends and collaborators was a remarkable man, Désiré Magloire Bourneville, fifteen years his junior, who is one of the savants depicted in the famous picture Brouillet made of Charcot demonstrating a case of hysteria in a patient being held up by Babinski. Primarily attached to the Bicêtre as an attending physician, Bourneville maintained the closest contact with La Salpêtrière as one of the authors of the *Iconographie Photographique* mentioned earlier in this chapter. A pioneer in medical photography, he edited the *Revue photographique des hôpitaux*. As an enthusiastic writer and propagandist, Bourneville was particularly concerned with improvement of hospitals and asylums. He sought to have these services divorced from the church and taken over by the state or municipality. But his appetite for work seems to have been insatiable. In 1873, he founded *Le progrès médical*, which became a journal of prestige and importance. In 1880, he took on the editorship of the new *Archives de neurologie*, whose appearance indicated yet again that neurology had come of age. The author of the book *Science et miracle*, he also edited a series of monographs published from the office of *Le progrès médical*. These include a translation of Johann Weier's famous book as well as books on witchcraft, faith healing, demonic possession, and similar topics. These works seem now to

71

be little known (even in France), but they are of the greatest interest because in several cases contemporary documents are presented together with very perceptive editorials. The series was called the *Collection Bourneville*, or *Bibliothèque Diabolique* (see appendix). It was Bourneville who was so impressed by Charcot's earliest lectures that he chose to edit and arrange them for publication, a task that eventually culminated in the *Oeuvres complètes*.

In his lectures Charcot constantly gave attention to the signs that distinguish a genuine hysterical symptom from the product of conscious simulation. This was most necessary, for his English contemporary Sir Horatio Donkin wrote as late as 1892 :

> The steps from the lowest to the highest grade of hysteria are imperceptible and the intermixture of imposture is often hard to recognize or duly appreciate. This difficulty has given rise to the common error of regarding hysterical disorder as deliberate sham and thus limiting its sphere to the extent of rendering the subject unintelligible.[24]

In 1873 Charcot resumed his lectures which, as he said, had been rudely interrupted two years earlier (by the siege of Paris) and chose as his subject an uncommon form of the great neurosis, namely 'hysterical ischuria.' This condition is so rare as to have its existence doubted and involves a failure in excretion of fluid that would be incredible except for the fact that it is accompanied by excessive vomiting of an aqueous solution of urea. Introducing a case of ischuria, Charcot spoke of 'his master Rayer, who never lost an opportunity of expatiating at length on the various deceptions of which hysterical patients are guilty.'[25] Charcot admitted that he had been incredulous regarding ischuria, but his opinion was modified by the case now presented. He gave a word on

> . . . *simulation*, which is met with at every step in the history of hysteria. One finds oneself acknowledging the amazing craft, sagacity and perseverance which women . . . especially under the influence of this great neurosis . . . will put in play . . . especially when a physician is to be the victim. But it does not seem to me that the erratic paruria of hysteria has ever been shown to be

wholly simulated. Though they [the women] certainly take pleasure in distorting, by exaggerations, the principal circumstances of their disorder, in order to make them appear extraordinary and wonderful.[26]

Charcot sketched out the sequence of events in fraudulent cases. They started with mild symptoms (some urinary retention, some vomiting) that though genuine aroused special interest. This interest encouraged the patient to amplify the marvellousness of the condition, and liquid would emerge from ears or nose. Charcot quoted the history of Joséphine Roulier, in whose case a strait-jacket had proved a very effective cure. Some pellets of hard matter were found hidden in the bed ready for use. With his own patient, Charcot had ensured that she was watched by two devoted patients of his own. 'The best possible police, women over women, for you are aware that if women enter into any plot between themselves they rarely succeed.'[27] This patient's fluid intake was carefully logged and correlated quantitatively with the amount of fluid lost by vomiting, and the real and non-fraudulent nature of the ischuria was established beyond doubt. Charcot stressed that in this patient's case, as in others, there was little doubt that the ischuria, once shown to be genuine, could be inferred to be hysterical for there was no failure of general health as would inevitably occur with an excretory block of organic origin. In fact, as with astasia-abasia (already noted), the general healthiness of hysterics was a regular and notable feature, and as such it was a valuable aid in differential diagnosis.

Charcot also insisted that hysteria was not usually monosymptomatic. For example, his ischuric patient had been in the Salpêtrière four years, having a history of convulsions and now a vast permanent contracture of the left side, ovarian pain, and complete hemianesthesia of the entire left half of the face and body. Charcot believed that in hysteria an anesthesia of some part of the integument was likely to be found if looked for. Janet and others admitted this, but claimed the frequency was lower than Charcot thought.[28] Some writers have suggested that Charcot asserted that anesthesia is invariably a feature of hysteria. But this is quite untrue; he maintained only that it occurred frequently. Janet agreed that in two-thirds of hysterics

c* 73

anesthesia accompanies the other hysterical symptoms. Now, it is possible for a patient to be quite unaware that he is anesthetic in some area of his skin. Consequently, the discovery of such an area tends to exculpate him from the charge that he is simulating some other and more prominent symptom. The matter, of course, is not quite so simple as this, because of the possibility that the very search for anesthetic patches when instituted by the physician may lead to their production in the hysteric by an innocent process of unconscious reaction to such a suggestion. (However, this very suggestibility is in itself a feature of the acute hysterics, so that the end result—diagnostically—is not much different, as will be discussed in the sequel.)

Charcot regarded the incidence of anesthesia and sensory disturbances of vision as so useful diagnostically (both in respect of the problem of fraud and for distinguishing the hysterical from the organic) that he called these signs the stigmata of hysteria. Janet says jocularly:

> Well, Charcot nearly brought us back to the time of the celebrated inquisitor Bodin, and, in our clinics, we are somewhat like the woman who sought for witches. We blindfold the subject, we turn his head away, rub his skin with our nail, prick it suddenly with a hidden pin, watch his answers or starts of pain; the picture has not changed.[29]

But Janet agreed that the anesthesia of Charcot must remain in practice a very important stigma, the search for which remained in the first rank of the methods of diagnosis.

Charcot also impressed on his students that disturbances of vision of which the patient was generally unaware occurred sometimes in isolation from skin anesthesia, but frequently in association with either total anesthesia (involving the whole body surface) or with hemianesthesia. As an example of the latter, he demonstrated a girl with deep anesthesia involving not only the skin but the muscles and nerve tracts on the whole of the left side of her body. On the anesthetized side there was also a diminution of taste, hearing, and smell; a loss of visual acuity; a reduction in color perception; and a shrinkage of the visual field. In most cases the shrinkage of the field of vision is concentric, the center

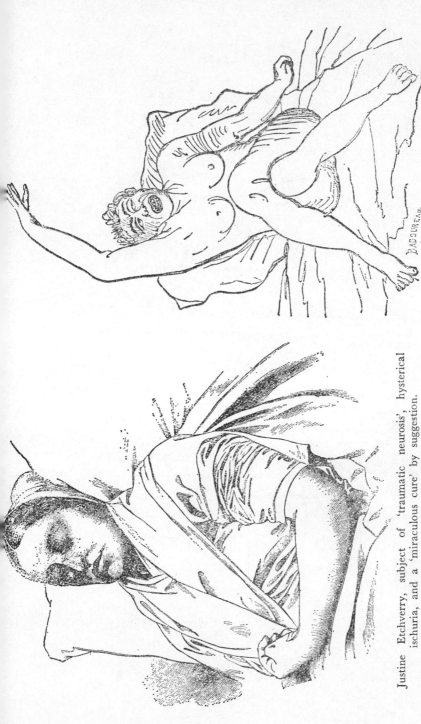

Justine Etchverry, subject of 'traumatic neurosis', hysterical
ischuria, and a 'miraculous cure' by suggestion.

Hysterical attack as 'traumatic neurosis'. (From *Clinical Lectures I*)

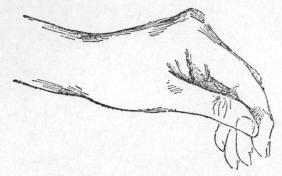

Hysterical contracture of the left hand.

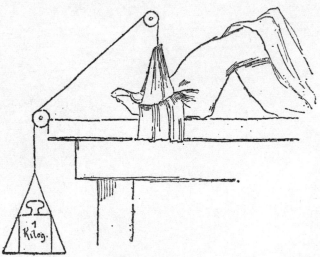

Experiment intended to verify the reality of the
contracture of the hand.
(From *Clinical Lectures III*)

of the field being normal and the periphery contracted within normal limits. Patients can be quite unaware of this contraction, particularly when it relates to one eye only. But the patient can be unaware of this condition even when both eyes show a considerable restriction of the visual field. Janet remarked:

This is a curious fact to which I remember having attracted the attention of Charcot, who had not remarked it, and was very much surprised at it. I showed him two of our young patients playing very cleverly at ball in the courtyard of La Salpêtrière. Then, having brought them before him, I remarked to him that their visual field was reduced to a point, and I asked him whether he would be capable of playing at ball, if he had before each eye a card merely pierced with a small hole.[30]

It was, of course, very remarkable indeed and tells us much about the nature of hysteria. But we shall return to this phenomenon later.

Permanent contracture of a muscle giving rise to a permanently bent wrist, elbow, knee, or pelvic joint is, of course, something the patient cannot be unaware of. How is it to be distinguished from a consciously willed and maintained contracture? Charcot reminded his class of the simple observation that a hysterical permanent contracture is maintained during sleep and that it disappears or relaxes only under chloroform anesthesia, which, on occasion, has to be very deep. But Charcot was interested in illuminating more clearly the distinction between voluntary and involuntary contraction and therefore improvised his own method of 'lie detection.' If a limb was being held in a contracted position, a reaction drum with a tracing mechanism was connected to it to record minute movements made by the limb. In addition, the respiration rate was recorded by a pneumograph attached to the chest. In one demonstration two subjects were compared: a robust and vigorous man with no symptoms (one of the clerical staff at the Salpêtrière), and a slight and delicate girl of sixteen years—a hysteric with sensory hemianesthesia and an anesthesia on the left side. Her left hand had a permanent contracture maintained during sleep, the thumb being bent over toward the palm. This thumb was put into a little sling attached to a loaded pulley. In the course of a half-hour, the thumb became gradually raised under the effect of the traction. When released from the sling the thumb returned to its original bent position without any appearance of fatigue in the hand or arm of the patient. The pneumograph record showed that the breathing remained even and regular, and the pressure drum showed no tremulousness. The experiment was repeated with the healthy young man. His thumb gradually yielded, though hardly any sooner than the girl's. However, his respiration chart soon became very disordered, displaying a jagged curve, and the pressure drum also registered marked fluctuations.

Charcot sometimes demonstrated patients in whom simulation could be recognized. As he pointed out, 'the desire to deceive even without purpose, by a kind of disinterested worship of art for art's sake, though sometimes with the idea of creating a sensation, to excite pity, is a common enough experience, particularly in hysteria.'[31] Noting that a patient sometimes does create all at once an imaginary group of symptoms, he also pointed to cases in which dissimulation acts merely so as to exaggerate real symptoms. For example, Charcot introduced his class to Mlle A, a fifteen-year-old girl from St Petersburg suffering from facial spasm. For comparison he brought in a patient aged fifty, a hysteric of long standing with stigmata in addition to a hysterical facial tic, which expressed itself in frequent spontaneous paroxysms—a rapid blinking and quivering of the eye—for which no means of suppression could be found. In little Mlle A, however, the spasms were completely inhibited by a pad on the right eye. When the pad was raised, a contraction of the muscles on the right side of the face resulted. If the eye remained entirely uncovered, spasm occurred more energetically still, with a frightful distortion and fixed expression of the countenance. Charcot recounted A's history as follows.

It had begun a year earlier, with spasm of the muscles of the orbit of the eye only. Next there was a period of attacks of the 'hystericks'—laughing, crying, shouting, and finally the spasm of the whole face. Spasms of both eye and face are common enough in hysterical subjects, Charcot remarked, but in A's case his suspicions were aroused by the facts that (1) the inhibitory pressure of the pad was extremely slight, and (2) the pad was efficacious only if applied by the doctors but not when put on by A herself. Charcot believed that the eye muscle spasm was a genuine symptom, but that the grimace of the lower face was an elaboration—superadded, invented, simulated. Why? He suggested the pleasure resulting from a love of notoriety, the satisfaction of deceiving not only her elders and betters but eminent physicians also and lastly the grand tour of Europe for consulting the *médecins* of Vienna, Paris, and London. Here Charcot adumbrates one of the features of neuroses—the secondary gain —as Freud called it. His opinion was confirmed by a simple experiment.

Mlle A was observed with her eyelids uncovered. She soon became very fatigued. After fifteen minutes she was breathless and in a cold sweat, and a nervous storm seemed imminent. After four weeks of treatment by isolation from her family, as well as by employment of various techniques such as application of magnets and static electricity (routine at the Salpêtrière), she was cured except for occasional spasms of the eye only.

In presenting a case of hysterical mutism, Charcot thought it his duty to point out that hysterical mutes were often very unjustly treated and thought to be simulators or malingerers. This was very serious in the army or for persons under criminal charges; they were often dealt with barbarously. For example, electric shocks were often applied to the larynx, a practice of some danger. It is however fairly easy, Charcot insisted, to distinguish the genuinely afflicted from the fraud:

Very few simulators have the intelligence to combine and display, with the object of deceit, all the symptoms that belong to the natural history of hysterical mutism, without taking from or adding in any way to this group of symptoms, at once so special and so complex.[32]

The malingerer was usually betrayed by overelaboration. Charcot quoted, as a fictitious example of a simulator, Lucinda in Molière's *Le médecin malgré lui,* who pointed to her head, mouth, and chin and uttered monosyllables 'Han, hi, hon, han.' The legitimate mute, however, remains silent, and if he makes a gesture, it is toward his throat where he believes the obstacle to be.

Charcot recounted an experience to show that even when simulation seems very plausible, in reality the symptoms may be perfectly genuine. With Professor Brouardel he examined Hélène, a twenty-four-year-old prisoner accused of infanticide, the actual fact of the killing not being in question. On arrest she lost her speech after the first interrogation. But Charcot and Brouardel rejected the obvious interpretation that this was voluntary. Hélène was totally mute without any sound or gesture, but had complete general anesthesia with retraction of the visual field. One fact was absolutely peremptory : The patient wrote fluently and accurately, and in this way confessed her crime. A malingerer would have refused to write.

In Charcot's day, the expansion of industry and the increasing organization of the working class engendered new medico-legal problems in the sphere of industrial compensation for injury. Similarly, as the railways spread across Europe and North America, railway accidents became a prolific source of legal claims from members of the general public. A condition resulting from train crashes became known as 'railway spine.' Charcot called it a very practical question; 'millions of dollars' hung in the scale by way of disputed damages throughout the world.[33] Frequently, these were cases of hysteria—'obstinate states that present themselves after accidents and render the victims incapable of moving for months and years. It is very often hysteria and nothing but this.' Charcot showed, as we shall see, that nervous troubles often derived from the 'psycho-nervous commotion' even when the victim sustained little or no physical injury. These disorders were undoubtedly produced or occasioned by the accident, even if their appearance was delayed. It is clear that the question of malingering was vital to the medico-legal situation, as it became in wartime. Apropos of World War I, Professor Chavigny said that the exceptional emotional tone of the war had occasioned numerous hysteric crises, and that these had been interpreted quite wrongly as malingering which merited court martial. He added :

We observed very carefully and impartially a series of cases and in spite of all to the contrary, we are convinced of the clinical existence of true hemianaesthesia or anaesthesia of the limbs according to Charcot's descriptions.[34]

Professor Chermitte remarked:

The examinations we performed on hundreds of soldiers during the war have proved in the most striking manner that many patients, who previously had never been examined medically, exhibit in one or another region of the body a loss of sensation to pain to such a degree that we could insert long needles through their arms or legs without their giving any evidence of the slightest feeling of pain.[35]

In the *Éloge de J.-M. Charcot* pronounced at the Sorbonne in 1925, Pierre Marie declared:

But what dominates the work of Charcot on hysteria, that will never perish and will continue to serve as a guide to future medical generations, was his demonstration of hysteria in the male. . . . How valuable were the teachings of Charcot for all those physicians and surgeons who, twenty years after his death . . . had to give their advice on so many cases [of traumatic hysteria]. How valuable too were his teachings for the experts who, during the war, were faced with the dual responsibility of maintaining an equitable balance between the State and those who fought for it![36]

Some writers subsequent to Lepois had noted male hysterics or admitted the theoretical possibility of hysteria in men. But in 1892, Charcot could still write with accuracy that,

As regards sex, the unanimous opinion until a few years ago, was that hysteria is essentially and exclusively peculiar to the female sex and . . . its etymological derivation has greatly contributed to perpetuate this view. It is known as synonymous with *furor uterinus* in all classes of society, even among physicians. This however is a mistake.[37]

The honor for definitely establishing that hysteria occurs in men was Briquet's and rests on his studies in the Paris hospitals.

According to his treatise of 1859, male hysterics were to be found, though only one-twentieth as often as women patients. The Salpêtrière, however, making a determined attack on the problem, discovered by means of its vastly improved diagnostic methods, that male admissions actually exceeded female ones. The reason for this excess of male patients lay in the large number of hysterical working-men admitted. In the upper classes, Charcot said, female cases still exceeded male cases, 'a fact probably due to the rareness of traumatism and intoxication, which in the poorer classes are, par excellence, the exciting causes of hysteria.[38]

Similarly, according to Freud, 'certain conditions which had been ascribed to alcohol or lead poisoning were hysterical.'[39] By *trauma* we can mean either an actual injury, or the psychological shock or fright involved when an accident or other violence occurs or is threatened. Alcoholism, of course, often involves accident or violence as well as delirium, and many of the alcoholics proved in fact to be traumatic hystericals.

The news from the Salpêtrière was slow of acceptance abroad. Freud spent a year with Charcot and returned to Vienna in 1886. Reporting to the Gesellschaft der Aerzte (Medical Society) upon what he had learned, he was met coldly. Bamberg, the chairman, said it was incredible. Meynert urged him to find male hysterics in Vienna, but the senior physicians were unhelpful. One of them declared it was nonsense, '*Hysteron* (sic) means the uterus. So how can a man be hysterical?' Producing at last a male hemianesthesiac for inspection, Freud was politely applauded, but all interest in him was dropped.[40] Freud does not mention it, but the oddest fact about the Viennese attitude is this: In 1881, Rosenthal, Professor of Nervous Diseases at Vienna, had published an excellent review of hysteria, giving all Briquet's statistics—with a preface by Charcot![41]

The belief in the restriction of hysteria to women did not rest entirely upon that sex's unique endowment with the uterus. Hippocrates had indicated that hysteria occurs in women suffering from sexual deprivation and advised marriage as a cure. Many doctors echoed this advice, often with disastrous results, though—of course—with some successes. Theophrastus Bombastus von Hohenheim, that is to say, Paracelsus ('greater than Celsus') had described hysteria as a *chorea lasciva*. In the nineteenth century, many textbooks associated hysteria in women with lewd thoughts and wanton inclinations. As Janet humorously put it:

> It was the fashion for a certain time to say that hysteria was a very rare disease; you know that it had a bad reputation, that a kind of dishonour attached to this word, and that people tried to persuade themselves that this shameful disease was not of frequent occurrence. By a kind of international irony, people were willing to admit, after the innumerable studies made by French physicians, that hysteria was frequent only among French women, which astonished nobody, on account of their bad reputation. . . . If the hysterical seemed to be less numerous in other countries, it is first because physicians did not recognize them, then because they would not give them their real appellation. When medical instruction is more general in this matter, when prejudices have vanished, it will probably be acknowledged that in this matter, as in many others, the other nations have no reason for envying France.[42]

Freud says somewhere in his writings that at the Salpêtrière under Charcot, the master so disapproved of the supposed associations of sexuality with hysteria that all the pupils and the staff, like the patients, regarded it as an insulting suggestion. In his 1892 *Dictionary* article Charcot wrote:

> As to sexual life, we protest against the opinion universally adopted by the public that all hysterical women have a tendency to lubricity, almost bearing on nymphomania. Far from this, our opinion founded on the observation of numerous hysterical females in the Salpêtrière is, that hysterical women are less sexual than sane and normal individuals; we may even add that hysterical patients with total anesthesia show absolute indifference to intercourse. Hysterical men as well as women often form love-plots and write amatory letters, but as regards the act itself they do not show the sexuality generally attributed to them; some are affected with *spermatorrhoea* which is closely allied to impotence.[43]

Charcot chose to be guided by the facts of observation which he mentions together with the discovery made at the Salpêtrière that a large proportion of hysterias in both men and women follow on traumatic experiences. Thus there was no warrant for supposing that sexual drives were the essential cause of hysteria. At the same time, it is worth attending to some of Freud's reminiscences:

> While I was writing my *History of the Psycho-Analytic Movement* in 1914 there occurred to my mind some remarks made to me by Breuer, Charcot and Chrobak [an eminent Viennese gynaecologist], which might have led me to the discovery earlier [i.e., of sexuality as frequently a causative agency in hysteria]. But at the time I did not understand what these authorities meant; *indeed they had told me more than they knew themselves or were prepared to defend.* What I had learned from them lay dormant and passive within me, until the chance of my cathartic experiments brought it out as an apparently original discovery.[44]

The paper Freud refers to provides an interesting sidelight on Charcot's personality.

> At one of Charcot's evening receptions [in 1885], I happened to be standing near the great teacher at a moment when he appeared to be telling Brouardel some very interesting story from his day's work. I hardly heard the beginning, but gradually my attention was seized by what he was saying. A young married couple from the Far East: the woman a confirmed invalid, the man either impotent or exceedingly awkward. '*Tâchez donc,* I heard Charcot repeating, *je vous assure, vous y arriverez.*' Brouardel, who spoke less loudly, must have expressed his astonishment that symptoms such as the wife's could have been produced in such circumstances. For Charcot suddenly broke in with great animation, '*Mais, dans des cas pareils c'est toujours la chose génitale, toujours . . . toujours . . . toujours*'; and he crossed his arms over his stomach, hugging himself and jumping up and down on his toes several times in his own characteristic lively way. I know that for one second I was almost paralyzed with amazement and said to myself, 'Well, but if he knows that, why does he never say so?'[45]

Freud did not question Charcot as to the knowledge obtained from the *secrets d'alcôve* (Breuer's phrase), because all his available interest was absorbed in the work on brain anatomy and hysterical paralyses he was doing during his year at La Salpêtrière. He says:

I have certainly not disclosed the illustrious parentage of this scandalous idea in order to saddle others with the responsibility for it. I am well aware that it is one thing once or twice, or even oftener, to fit words to an idea that comes in the form of a fleeting inspiration, and quite another to intend it seriously, to take it literally, to pursue it in spite of all difficulties into every detail and to win it a place among accepted truths. It is the difference between a casual flirtation and solemn matrimony with all its duties and difficulties.[46]

Zilboorg said (though in a different context) that Charcot's psychological intuition was always greater and truer than his official views on psychological reactions.[47] However this may have been, whether constrained by either scientific reluctance not to theorize beyond the facts, unconscious repression, or a kind of political tact, Charcot took care to say nothing to encourage the crude equation of hysteria with nymphomania. When lecturing on 'ovarian pain,' Charcot goes to great lengths not to be misunderstood. In some patients, he said, hemianesthesia somewhat paradoxically was found associated with ovarian hyperesthesia, that is, the surface of the abdomen in that region was hypersensitive. He had verified that in some patients this region was a *hysterogenic point*; pressure on it would engender the sensation of the hysterical aura. Charcot had also discovered that sometimes compression of this region could arrest even very violent hysterical attacks. This had been denied by Briquet, whose otherwise excellent book had one weak side: All that related to the ovary and uterus was treated 'in a spirit which seems singular in a physician.' Charcot regarded this as 'an unaccountable sentimentality, a kind of prudery.' It appeared as though the author's mind was always preoccupied by one dominant idea, for Briquet had said: 'In attempting to attribute everything to the ovary and uterus, hysteria is made a disorder of lubricity, a shameful affection, which is calculated to render hysterical patients objects of loathing and pity.'[48] Charcot said firmly that he himself was far from believing that lubricity is always at work in hysteria; he was even convinced of the contrary. Nor was he a partisan of the old doctrine, which taught that the source of all hysterias resides in the genital organs. But Charcot did believe it to be demonstrated that the ovary plays an important part in a special type of hysteria—the 'ovariform.' To prove his point, he presented to his class five patients with *ovarie*. Returning to the *convulsionnaires*, he censured Hecquet for suggesting that the *secours* was required by 'lubricity.'[49] 'For my own part I do not well understand what lubricity could have to do with blows of pestles and andirons administered with extreme violence, though I am far from forgetting what a depraved taste may give birth to.' While Charcot would not turn his face from an empirical fact, he would however do nothing to assist the notion of hysteria as a 'shameful affection.'[50]

We can allow Freud to summarize these aspects of Charcot's work in the discovery of the neuroses:

He began to turn his attention almost exclusively to hysteria, thus suddenly focussing general attention on this subject. This most enigmatic of all nervous diseases—no workable point of view having yet been found from which physicians could regard it— had just at this time come very much into discredit, and this ill-repute related not only to the patients but was extended to the physicians who treated this neurosis. The general opinion was that anything might happen in hysteria; hysterics found no credit whatsoever. First of all Charcot's work restored dignity to the subject; gradually the sneering attitude, which the hysteric could reckon on meeting when she told her story, was given up; she was no longer a malingerer, since Charcot had thrown the whole weight of his authority on the side of the reality and objectivity of hysterical phenomena. Charcot had repeated on a small scale the act of liberation commemorated in the picture of Pinel which adorned the lecture hall of the Salpêtrière.[51]

CHAPTER IV

The Causes of Hysteria

CHARCOT IS sometimes criticized for having drawn attention to the ovarian region and thereby having encouraged, it is alleged (even though unwillingly), the practice of surgical removal of the ovary in some hysterical patients.[1] But this criticism is more than a little misconceived, and Janet's opinion is the true one:

> You must be able quickly to recognise this disease, in order to foresee its evolution, to provide against its dangers, and immediately to begin a rational treatment. This early diagnosis is much more important still from another point of view; it will keep you . . . from making blunders. It is perhaps not very serious not to recognise a hysterical symptom and not to treat it; but what is always very serious is to mistake a hysterical symptom for another one, and to treat it for what it is not. You cannot imagine the medical blunders, and too often also the medical crimes, committed in this way. One of the greatest difficulties in the medical art and one of the greatest misfortunes of patients is that the hysterical diseases are only well characterized from the moral point of view, which usually is not examined at all; that they are very badly characterized from the physical point of view, and that they are uncommonly similar to all kinds of medical or surgical affections, for which they are easily mistaken. . . . Then the physician interposes, frightens the family, agitates the patient to the uttermost, and prescribes extraordinary diets, perturbing the life and exhausting the strength of the sick person. Finally, the surgeon is called in. Do not try to count the number of arms cut off, of muscles of the neck incised for cricks, of bones broken

for mere cramps, of bellies cut open for phantom tumours, and especially of women made barren for pretended ovarian tumours.

Humanity ought indeed to do homage to Charcot for having prevented a greater depopulation.[2]

Charcot was most appreciative of advances in surgery and rejoiced in the advent of neurosurgery for removal of brain tumors and correction of Jacksonian epilepsy, as well as in all the other legitimate operations of the surgeon. But he was well aware of the surgeon's neurosis—*mania operativa activa*. This mania was very rife in the nineteenth century, the era of the 'heroic surgeon.' Axel Munthe narrates his anxiety on being sent home from Chamonix with both legs severely crushed after he had fallen off the slopes of Mont Blanc. He was cared for by Professor Tillaux at the Hôtel-Dieu who forebore to amputate, but Munthe claimed to tremble at the thought of what would have happened to him had he fallen into the hands of one of the other leading surgeons of Paris.

Old Papa Richet [*not* Charles Richet] would have made me die of gangrene or blood poisoning; it was his speciality, rampant all over his medieval clinic. The famous Professor Péan, the terrible butcher of Hôpital St Louis, would have chopped off both my legs and thrown them on the heap of limbs on the floor of the amphitheatre. . . .[3]

This may be correct as applying to the operative mania. But for the year in question, which (so far as one can be sure with Munthe, who was not very strong on dates) was 1891, the aspersion is probably anachronistic in respect of surgical asepsis. Semmelweis had long been vindicated, and it was almost a quarter of a century since Lister had proposed his reforms. Munthe is probably repeating anecdotes relating to the surgery of two decades earlier.

Hysterical pain in the knee joint or the hip joint, said Charcot in one of his lectures, was often confused with that due to an organic cause. But absence of a material lesion was sufficiently demonstrated by the unprogressive nature of the malady and by the negative findings in autopsies. There were also biopsies, usually unintentional.

By a singular coincidence, the patients attacked with this affection clamour loudly for active surgical intervention, and thus . . . when these patients attacked with a *mania operativa passiva* find themselves unfortunately in the presence of surgeons affected with an analogous though active madness, *mania operativa activa*, the most fantastic operations can result, even amputations. For example the London physician Coulson quotes the case of a young girl who had a flexure of the knee with unbearable pain. A surgeon was at last found willing to amputate. Examination of the knee joint revealed normal and healthy nerve, muscle and tissue.[4]

One of the earliest distinctions successfully drawn at the Salpêtrière was between the epileptic seizure and the major hysterical attack. Although the latter might be colored by unconscious imitation of the epileptic fit, clear-cut differences emerged if observations were made with sufficient care and patience. The epileptic fit came on more suddenly; the patient was likely to fall and injure himself, uttering a peculiar cry. He lay prostrate, without struggling and with only minor and restricted movements. There was no speech; at most sighs and groans. Epileptic attacks were rare, but if repeated in short succession they generated a rise in temperature, with a marked deterioration of the patient's mental condition. The epileptic had no hysterical stigmata. His attacks could be inhibited to some extent by administration of bromide.

By contrast, the hysterical attack gave warning of its onset through the hysterical aura. The hysterical patient tended therefore to be lying down by the time that the attack started. Thus he avoided injury and, unlike the epileptic, tended to be unscarred. When the attack came on, he gave at most a feeble cry. However, his struggles were violent and often he had to be held down. He uttered exclamations and often intelligible words and phrases. Hysterical attacks could follow one another without intermission, perhaps scores of attacks in one day. Yet the health of the patient remained mysteriously unimpaired. His temperature stayed normal during any attack, however violent. No series of attacks, however dramatic or numerous, entailed any intellectual impairment. Bromides, though harmless, were of no effect in suppressing attacks. The patient had very frequently the stigmata of hysteria.[5]

The work was complicated by the fact that some of the epileptics were also hysterical, and much care was needed at first to distinguish the character of each attack experienced by these unfortunates. Because the hysterical attack mimicked the epileptic attack, Charcot originally applied to it the term *hystero-epilepsy*, but this designation eventually fell into disuse and was replaced by *major hysteria*, to distinguish it from the nonconvulsive forms. The distinction between the epileptic and the hysteric fit was for a long time, says Janet, considered impossible until settled by the 'School of the Salpêtrière.'[6]

In respect of paralyses and contractures, Charcot listed seven features associated with those of the hysterical kind which tended to enable their differential diagnosis from those of organic origin: (1) general health of the patient and of the affected limbs; (2) disappearance under chloroform; (3) association with hysterical attacks; (4) absence of temperature elevation; (5) distribution of pain; (6) association with other hysterical stigmata; and (7) sudden onset or relief.[7]

Charcot drew special attention to the fact that both a paralyzed limb and one in permanent contracture tended to remain strong. There was, of course, some atrophy or wastage (a very significant fact, when we consider the history of faith cures and 'miracles'), but in the hysterical paralysis or contracture it was usually much less pronounced than in similar disorders of organic cause. The general health of the patient also tended to be good. Moreover, in some cases the patients, instead of being depressed, worried, or anxious about their chronic illness, exhibited calmness, placidity, and—indeed—cheerfulness. Charcot christened this detachment *la belle indifférence*, a phrase that has lasted.

The persistence of hysterical contractures during sleep, albeit with some degree of relaxation, is diagnostic against conscious simulation as we have seen. The occurrence of some relaxation in sleep is, of course, diagnostic against organic causation. The finding is made certain by the tendency of the contracture to resolve completely under chloroform. Strikingly, hysterical contractures reappear immediately on the return of consciousness.[8]

88

Hysterical paralyses and contractures were often discovered to be the sequel to an earlier history of hysterical attacks. Occasionally, a paralysis would be lifted or a contracture resolved at the end of an attack. One patient 'Pin.,' whom Charcot introduced to his class, was freed of a flaccid paralysis of his left arm after a hysterical attack that had been induced by pressure at a hysterogenic point.

In organically determined conditions of rigidity or stiffness of joints, there was usually some slight local heating. This was not found in hysterical symptoms, where also the associated pain—if any—as reported by the patient differed in its provenance and subjective description from that experienced in organic affections.

Anesthesias found in any part of the body naturally added to the presumption of hysteria. But often they occurred in and around the contracted or paralyzed limb, or the hand, arm, or leg concerned in spasmodic or choreic movement. Thus a subject of Janet's who used to turn his right hand in a circle and make a see-saw movement with his right foot was almost insensible on the whole of the right side.[9] The subject in such a condition does not feel that he is making the movements, but thinks of it as if someone else was seizing his hand and turning it.

Anesthesia was still more characteristic of paralyses. Of course there are anesthesias associated with organic paralyses. Thus in tabes, the symptom that Charcot was the first to describe and which he called the *tabetic mask*, involves a loss of sensibility of part of the face. The patients are acutely aware of this loss and say that it gives them a horrible feeling. But hysterics who have facial anesthesia (and they are legion, says Janet) are either unaware or indifferent. Janet's brother, Jules, while an intern at La Pitié (almost adjoining La Salpêtrière on the west side) observed an interesting case.[10] A young lady had cut her wrist after falling through a glass door. A few days after the accident, the wound was healing well and there was no paralysis. She complained of a certain numbness, but more particularly was concerned about a persistent insensibility in the palm of the hand which was, in fact, associated with a severing of the median nerve and its superficial branches. But when the Janets examined her, they made the singular discovery that she had a hysterical anesthesia of the entire left side of which she was totally unaware. When they teased her that she complained of an insensibility that affected only a small portion of the palm of her hand, but did not even notice the much larger insensibility of the whole of her left side, the girl looked surprised and abashed.

Babinski, Charcot's famous pupil, studied the involuntary muscular reflexes in organic and hysterical paralyses. In an organically determined situation (a failure of the nerves associated with the muscles in question, or in the corresponding brain tissue), some of the reflexes must also be impaired. For example, the tendon reflexes of elbow, wrist, knee and the Achilles tendon are suppressed in tabes and are exaggerated in the case of cerebral damage due to hemorrhage, or when there are lesions of the pyramidal tract. Usually, however, hysterics show no modification of ordinary reflexes even in limbs that are flaccidly paralyzed; nor are there any disturbances of the electrical reactions. Thus the reaction called the 'reaction of degeneration,' which can establish itself rapidly in certain instances of lesions of the medulla, does not exist in hysterical paralyses.

Babinski's 'sign' (announced in 1896) relates to cutaneous reflexes. In normal adults, if the ball of the foot is rubbed slightly with a pin, the toes bend together toward the sole of the foot. In lesions of the medulla, a raising and extension of the toes ensues consequent to this stimulus, but not in hysteria. Contraction of the muscles of the skin is absent in various organic disorders, but not in neurosis, when various cutaneous areas are excited. Similarly, the slightest disturbances in optical reflexes or in the phenomena of visual accommodation should alert the physician to search for the organic lesions of either tabes or syphilitic meningitis. Babinski also showed that in hysterical paralysis muscular tone tends to be preserved. He insisted correctly that certain unconscious movements occur in apparently paralyzed limbs. Janet stressed the analogy between this fact and the preservation of unconscious perception and sensation in spite of hysterical anesthesia, as exemplified by the boys playing at ball.[11]

In one series of lectures Charcot demonstrated a whole platoon of male hysterics not only to prove their existence, but

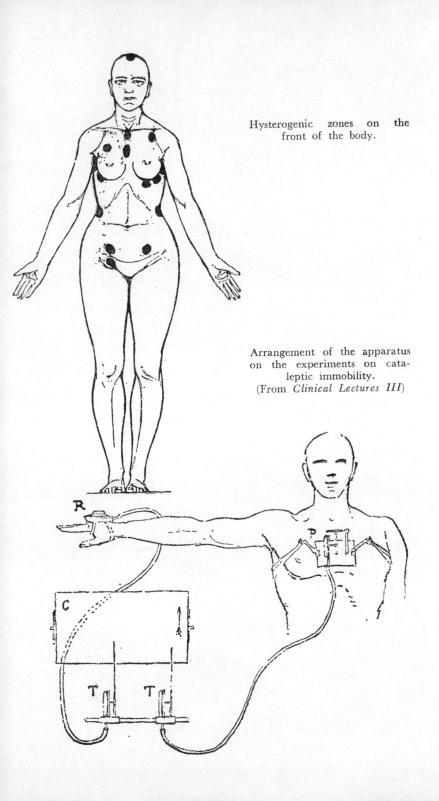

Hysterogenic zones on the
front of the body.

Arrangement of the apparatus
on the experiments on cataleptic immobility.
(From *Clinical Lectures III*)

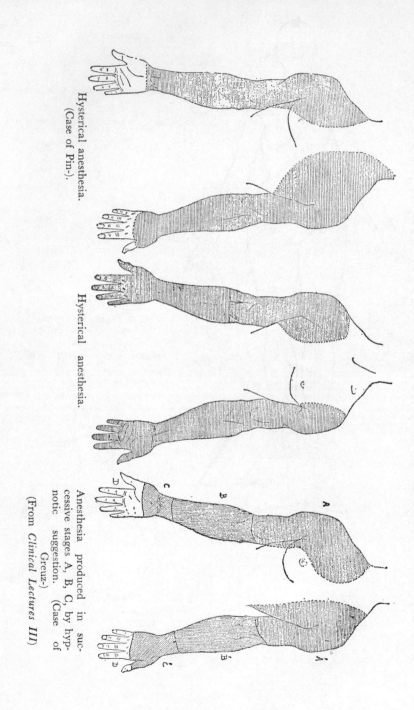

Hysterical anesthesia.
(Case of Pin-).

Hysterical anesthesia.

Anesthesia produced in successive stages A, B, C, by hypnotic suggestion. (Case of Greuz-)
(From *Clinical Lectures III*)

also to indicate many other points of interest. Among these hysterics were Pin., as aforementioned, and a young man called 'Porcz.,' whose right arm had a flaccid paralysis and was incapable of the slightest voluntary movement. The arm had a complete anesthesia that was not only cutaneous, but extended to deeper layers. However, Charcot pointed out, its distribution was quite different from the anesthesia due to nerve or brain lesions.[12] All the hysterical anesthesias of paralyzed limbs were complete, occupying a well-defined zone with a clear-cut circular edge to it. This was called *glove and sleeve anesthesia*; it was quite different from that due to lesions of the brain or the nerves: the radial, the median and the ulnar. Interruption of bounded by a clear-cut arc. Instead, it was very irregular and ragged. Spots of sensitivity were always mixed up with spots of anesthesia. This was so because the anesthesia was related to specific nerves that were either themselves disordered or radiated from the same specific sensory area of the brain.[13] Charcot used to say of hysterical anesthesia accompanying paralyses that it occurred in the form of 'geometric segments.'

These anesthesias therefore differ completely from those based on organic lesions. For instance, the hand has three principal nerves: the radial, the median and the ulnar. Interruption of one of these nerves produces a specific anesthesia whose distribution corresponds to the path of the nerve. Thus a lesion of the cubital nerve can produce insensitivity only in the little finger and in part of the fourth. Hysterical anesthesia of the hand involves the whole organ up to the wrist. Briquet was very puzzled by this lack of localization and wondered if it had something to do with the circulation of the blood, which, of course, it does not. In a word: Hysteria is ignorant of anatomy! This also illustrates a principle that Charcot stressed: Hysteria produces its symptoms in exaggerated form.

Similar considerations apply to the muscles of a paralyzed limb. Unless the whole relevant motor area of the cortex is defective, an organic nerve or brain lesion affects only some of the muscles, never all. Another rule that applies is that the parts of the body furthest from the brain cannot be less seriously affected than the nearer parts. Thus in organic cerebral paralysis of the leg, we cannot have more activity in the foot than in the thigh or the hip. Yet the reverse is frequently true in hysteria. There can be movement of the fingers on a paralyzed arm when the shoulder is absolutely immovable. Charcot, following the observations of Todd on paralysis of the leg, made a famous distinction between the *helicopode* and *helcopode* gaits. In the organic paralysis, the hip is usually relatively unimpaired; the patient can move it and uses it to perform the circular movement that carries the leg forward. In hysteria, the hip is immobile and consequently the leg must be dragged as an inert mass.[14]

In 1885 Freud, who had discerned that 'in the distance glimmered the great name of Charcot,' formed the plan of first obtaining an appointment as lecturer on nervous diseases in Vienna and of then going to Paris to continue his studies. The lectureship on Neuropathology to which he aspired came his way in the spring of that year, and in the autumn—assisted by a travelling fellowship—Freud made the journey to Paris where he stayed for a year, familiarizing himself with all that went on at the Salpêtrière. He says that Charcot 'was good enough to entrust me with the task of making a comparative study of organic and hysterical motor paralyses, based upon observations at the Salpêtrière. . . .'[15] But doubtless the program was assigned to him in a much more informal way. Freud as a youngster of twenty-nine, no doubt discussed this particular facet of neurology soon after his arrival and the 'Master,' having signified his general approval, the young physician 'from the Far East' (as Vienna was sometimes regarded by the scientific world of those days, so Freud remarks somewhere) was free to make as much use of the facilities as he could contrive. Elsewhere Freud says:

Before leaving Paris I discussed with the great man a plan for comparative study of hysterical and organic paralyses. I wished to establish the thesis that in hysteria paralyses and anaesthesia of the various parts of the body are dominated according to the popular idea of their limits and not according to anatomical facts.[16]

According to Freud, Charcot agreed with this view but was not really interested in penetrating more deeply into the psychology of the neuroses. Whether this assessment was accurate we will leave for later judgement. In any case, the finding that Freud formulated had already clearly emerged from the work at the Salpêtrière. As Janet put it :

> For the common people, the hand terminates at the wrist. They don't care if all the principal muscles that animate the hand and fingers are lodged beyond in the fore-arm. The hysteric person who paralyses her hand seems not to know that the immobility of her fingers is due in reality to a muscular disturbance in her fore-arm. She stops her anaesthesia at the wrist, as would the vulgar, who, in their ignorance say that if the hand does not move it is because the hand is diseased.[17]

Thus the way was open to a mental etiology for hysterias.

But Charcot traveled to the same conclusion by another route. As we shall see, he expressed it in a remarkably explicit way, using terminology that we tend to associate with his successors, Freud and Janet. Indeed, we are apt to credit the latter two with having invented the terms 'idea,' 'psychic,' 'unconscious,' 'ego,' and 'autosuggestion.' Charcot's own pronouncements seem to have been forgotten. Instead, prominence seems to be given to a remark to the effect that we have in hysteria 'what *for want of a better term* [italics supplied], we designate a *dynamical* or *functional lesion*.' This was apropos of the patient 'Porz.,' but may have been said on many occasions. Nowadays it seems to be held against Charcot, principally on the basis of his use of the word *lesion*. In ordinary usage *'lesion'* is a hurt, loss, or injury, but in pathology the word means any morbid change in function or structure of an organ or a tissue. There was in Charcot's time a rooted habit of thinking of a lesion primarily as a structural abnormality. But in 1867, it will be recalled, Charcot had remarked that the growth of biochemistry was leading pathologists to think also in terms of possible derangements of function which were structurally invisible, even under the technique of microhistology, but which were nonetheless real. These derangements were faults in metabolism and chemical reactions. They could occur within the cell or in ambient media, the circulating or diffusive fluids of the body. As electrophysiology advanced, it became clear that the electrical properties of nerve cells could contribute subtly to functional derangement.

Thus to some of Charcot's contemporaries, the terms 'dynamical' or 'functional lesion' could be understood in a fairly subtle way. But as Freud pointed out in 1893, chemical or electrochemical conditions of a kind leaving no trace after death might not be lesions in the old-fashioned sense, but were in fact organic lesions even though transitory. Freud pointed out that diffusive conditions of this kind, even though conceivably localized to restricted regions of the cerebral cortex, would produce paralyses resembling known organic paralyses.[18] It should be noted that Freud at no time accuses Charcot of limiting the functional lesion to chemical disturbances. Freud merely discusses in succession the various meanings readers could ascribe to Charcot's term. He does not claim to demonstrate what the functional lesion is, but merely to suggest a line of thought.

I will take the word 'functional or dynamic lesion' in its proper sense : 'alteration in function or mechanism.' Such an alteration, for example would be a diminution in excitability or in a physiological quality which in the normal state remains constant or varies within fixed limits. . . .

I will try to show that a functional alteration may exist without an accompanying organic lesion, at least without a lesion capable of detection even by means of the most delicate methods. In other words, I will give an appropriate example of a primary functional change; to do so I only ask permission to pass over into the field of psychology, which cannot be ignored in dealing with hysteria.

With Janet I maintain that it is the common, popular idea of the organs . . . that is at work in hysterical paralyses as well as in anaesthesias, etc. . . . The lesion of hysterical paralysis will be an alteration of the concept of the idea 'arm' for example. . . .

Psychologically considered the paralysis of the arm consists in the fact that the 'concept' arm cannot enter into association with those other ideas that make up the ego, of which the body of the individual is an important part. The lesion, then, would consist

94

in the abolition of the accessibility of the concept 'arm' in association.[19]

This example calls to mind Janet's description of people with hysterical paralyses. 'If you question such persons, you find that they seem not to have kept the remembrance of their limb, they do not know any longer what this paralyzed limb used to do and they can no longer make the efforts of imagination necessary to conceive it.'[20] Janet maintains that Charcot's pupil Féré was one of the first who insisted on this point. Writing in 1892, Féré said of a patient :

> After having shut her eyes, I ask her to try to represent to herself her left hand executing movements of extension and flexion. She is not able to do it. She can represent to herself her right hand making very complicated movements on the piano, but on her left, she has the sensation that her hand is lost in empty space. She cannot even represent to herself its form.[21]

It is clear from the way Freud developed the notion, that in speaking so circumspectly of a functional lesion, Charcot was keeping all options open. It would be interesting to have his reactions today to the unsolved but very active problem of schizophrenia. Freud and other workers thought of schizophrenia as primarily psychological. At present an intensive search is afoot for environmental causes. But chemical aspects are also much in favor, and a chemical or autointoxication theory clearly involves an organic lesion of a functional nature.[22] It is worth recalling Charcot's confession of faith in his 1867 lecture, when he spoke of the new medical outlook : 'It goes so far as to believe that vital properties will one day be combined with properties of a physical order : at least, it insists for the future that a correspondence, not an antagonism, must exist between these two forms of energy.'[23] If for *vital* we read *mental*, we see that Charcot's formulation of the 'functional lesion' was in fact within the terms of reference he had set himself many years before. If pressed, he might have said that psychology and brain function, though not simply reducible to each other, were nevertheless not antagonistic but in correspondence. As to the character of that correspondence, Charcot probably would have said in 1890 (as in 1867) that, beyond a certain point, Nature was deaf to our questions and would not answer them. Modern critics of Charcot's 'dynamical lesion,' who have failed to note how exquisitely noncommital he was, would do well to remember that in most of the questions concerning consciousness and the unconscious, Nature is still both deaf and mute.

Yet, as Freud says: 'Charcot was the first to teach us that we must turn to psychology for the explanation of the hysterical neurosis.'[24] These teachings emerged mainly from his researches into the onset of hysteria in individual patients. The onset of a paralysis, a contracture, or mutism was always abrupt when the condition was hysterical. With organic ailments, however, the onset was always slower, and the symptom itself was less intense and often accompanied by pain, yet pain was absent in the hysterical forms.

In the case of a paralysis or contracture setting in after an injury the distinction was, of course, not so obvious as with a condition coming on without prelude. But the distinction could be made. In patients with certain organic lesions such as cerebral or spinal sclerosis, the superaddition of a mild injury, blow, or electric shock or even blistering due to a medicated plaster could, said Charcot, produce paralyses or contractures. But these conditions came on much less suddenly than hysterical ones subsequent to an injury. Also, they were proportionate to the severity of the injury. Hysterical conditions could be wildly disproportionate and exaggerated in relation to the degree of injury. At one stage Charcot described this phenomenon in physiological terms as an 'exaggerated reflex excitability,' and gave Sir Benjamin Brodie the credit for noticing it as long ago as 1837, when he described a contracture of the arm following pricks of the fingers.

Charcot gave many illustrations of reflex excitability. He introduced to his class 'two young persons [exemplifying *la belle indifférence*] with a flippant air and a taste for finery rendered manifest by the ribbons and flowers with which they are adorned.' Both suffered from minor hysterical attacks, *ovarie*, and anesthesias. One girl had spontaneous contractures after her attacks. If small repeated taps were applied to the wrist of either, then the corresponding fingers would assume a position of exaggerated flexion and remain fixed for some hours. In another patient, faradization (i.e., a mild electric current) produced a partial ulnar deformity of the hand. Charcot never withdrew his postulate of 'reflex hyperexcitability.' Indeed, he demonstrated similar phenomena in hypnotized hysterics. But in parallel with the notion of hyperexcitability of muscular reflexes, he stressed the psychological aspects connected with the onset of hysterical symptoms.[25]

Charcot cited numerous examples of disproportion between the injury and consequent hysterical symptoms. Thus a girl of sixteen years received an infinitesimal cut on the arm which healed within five days. Yet a contracture of the hand set in, together with hemianesthesia and *ovarie*, still persisting a year after the accident. A vigorous blacksmith aged thirty-five, the father of a family, received a burn on the forearm. The wound healed. He had shown little emotion at the time of the accident. A few days later, his arm felt heavy with numbness in the fingers which developed into a hysterical contracture of the forearm gradually over seven weeks. Another patient, 'Rig.,' while at work was seriously frightened at the prospect of being crushed under a falling barrel. In the event he sustained only minor damage to the left hand. But ten days later an hysterical attack ensued. Rig. eventually became a chronic hysteric in the Salpêtrière. He had continual attacks with loss of consciousness, convulsions with great movements, and *attitudes passionelles*, during which he uttered gloomy words and had frightening visions.

Pin. (who has twice been mentioned) was a stonemason aged eighteen who sustained a slight bruise in a fall. Three days later, his left arm became partially paralyzed. Twenty-two days after the fall, the paralysis was complete. It had all characteristics of a hysterical paralysis, for ten months later, though the paralysis persisted, there was no atrophy nor were there any abnormal electrical reactions in the muscles. The patient Porcz., also referred to earlier, was a young coachman who had been thrown from the driving seat, falling on his right shoulder. There was some pain in the shoulder and arm but no bruising. He rested for five days after the accident. On the sixth day the arm became flaccid and quite incapable of movement.

Great interest attached to the patient 'Dum.,' a young man aged thirty. On breaking his arm he was, Charcot says, as if 'stunned' and some months after still had some amnesia relating to the accident. After the accident he had no experience of pain in the arm which 'seemed dead.' He was unable 'to feel the arm at all,' which seemed 'absent from shoulder to fingertips.' The limb was flaccid and without voluntary movement, but not stiff. Two days after the accident it was put into a plaster splint, which was eventually removed. Fifteen days after the removal of the splint the arm was found contracted into a flexed state, as if held in a sling. Under chloroform it was established that there was no physical deformity, and hence the condition was a spasmodic contracture. Charcot expressed the opinion that the moderate pressure of bandaging had stimulated the conversion of a hysterical paralysis into a contracture. Dum. improved under treatment. He decided to leave the hospital, but returned later after having consulted a Paris doctor who treated him by Dr Burq's method, which involved covering the patient's hands and fingers with plates and rings of copper (*metallotherapy*). Dum.'s hand remained deformed.

Charcot was so impressed by the occurrence of Dum.'s contracture, that he tried a simple experiment with a patient called 'Mouil.,' who had a flaccid paralysis of the arm. A bandage was applied and produced a complete contracture of the wrist and the fingers. The contracture disappeared completely on removal of the bandage.[26]

Charcot henceforth put less stress on reflex hyperexcitability and tended to shift the emphasis in paralysis to psychological aspects. In 1892 he wrote:

It seems probable that hystero-traumatic paralysis is, among others, formed by the following process: A man predisposed to hysteria has received a blow on the shoulder. This slight traumatism or local shock has sufficed to produce in this nervous individual a sense of numbness extending over the whole of the limb and a slight indication of paralysis. In consequence of this sensation the idea comes to the patient's mind that he might become paralysed; in one word through *autosuggestion*, the rudimentary paralysis becomes real.

98

In other words the phenomenon is brought about in the cerebral cortex, the seat of all psychical operations. The idea of movement, in the course of being executed, is already movement; the idea of absence of movement, if strong, is already the realization of motor-paralysis; all this is entirely in conformity with the laws of psychology. We know sufficiently from mental pathology that there are ideas so fixed that it becomes impossible for the patient to escape the obsession. However this may be, the different forms of hysterical paralysis present themselves in general with certain common characters of which one of the most typical is anaesthesia.[27]

The reader may be a little surprised to see how much Charcot had anticipated the ideas of later workers such as Janet. It is with Janet that we associate the term *autosuggestion*, and also the *idée fixe*—the fixed idea, as well as the essentially psychological interpretation. But almost all of this is to be found in Charcot's final pronouncements. In fairness we need to note that Janet came to the Salpêtrière in 1890, and it is possible that the exposition quoted above owes some aspects of its formulation and language to discussions between Charcot and Janet. But it needs also to be said that Charcot was saying very similar things at least as early as 1885, as we know from his lectures. It is worth noting also that Charcot no longer spoke in terms of the dynamic or functional lesion of the cortex, but only in terms of the cerebral cortex as the '*seat* of psychical operations.' We may recall that it was in the same article (signed by himself and Pierre Marie) that hysteria was spoken of as 'less a disease than a peculiarly constituted mode of feeling and reaction.'

Other cases also indicated to Charcot that 'The fright in accident is more important than the wound itself,' and 'Emotion plays a great part.' That is to say, trauma in its sense of 'shock' is more important than in its sense of physical injury. Indeed, there were occasions where the emotional side alone was all sufficing. Charcot quoted a wealth of cases in which 'shock' without injury precipitated hysteria. Of these he remarked: 'Nervous troubles often occur in such cases apart from any traumatic lesion, as a result of the *psycho-nervous* commotion, produced by, yet often not appearing immediately, after the accident.'[28]

Thus the patient 'Ler.,' an acute sufferer from *grande hystérie*, had a history of frightening experiences. At the age of eleven, she had been attacked by a mad dog; later, she was terrified by an unexpected sight of a corpse; and finally, she had an alarming confrontation with desperadoes. In the convulsive stage of her attacks she was prey to delirium, talking of being bitten and of 'villains, robbers, brigands.' Similarly, in the terminal phase of an attack she would hallucinate horrible animals, skeletons, and specters. Another patient, Justine 'Etch.,' had a paralysis of the left half of the body with a permanent contracture. Charcot describes her as intelligent and as having been a hospital nurse in the Basses-Pyrénées. She had enjoyed perfect health until the age of thirty-four, when she sustained what Charcot described as a 'violent moral shock' (presumably an attempted sexual assault) that precipitated her hysterical seizures.

A sixteen-year-old youth, described by Charcot as 'intelligent and with a joyous disposition, except for a tendency to fly into a rage,' and free from excessive timidity, was attacked in the street by two evildoers. He lost consciousness but had no trace of any wound. A fortnight later hysterical seizures set in, accompanied by patches of anesthesia and diminution of the field of vision.[29]

During a quarrel a stone was thrown at another patient, a young stonemason called 'Lys.' Although the projectile missed him, Lys. was severely frightened and convulsive attacks started fifteen days later, together with trembling of the limbs and chronic insomnia. Lys.'s case resembled that of 'Le Log.,' another celebrated patient of Charcot's, who developed hysteria thinking he had been wounded by a carriage that in fact did *not* run over him.[30]

Whether we should describe the causative agency as pure fright or more specifically as the expectation of a specific injury is, of course, a moot point. Janet gave an interesting case from his own observation, in which the hysterical symptom developed subsequent to a purely psychic trauma, but in accordance with the specific injury the patient *expected* to receive but which, in the concrete event, he escaped. A traveler by rail was imprudent enough to attempt changing carriages while the train was in motion. While he was on the step outside the train, he noticed that the train was about to enter a tunnel. Hanging on with his right hand and foot, he expected that his left side would be crushed against the arch of the tunnel. He fainted, but was hauled in, uninjured, by his traveling companions. Yet in due course, he developed a paralysis of the entire left side of the body.[31]

In other cases pure emotion, not specifically related to any defined localized physical injury, was found to have precipitated hysteria. Charcot's pupil Féré noted a girl patient who dreamt one night that she was pursued at high speed by a man through the streets of Paris until she was totally exhausted. The next day she was paralyzed.[32] Here it might be admitted that paralysis could be regarded as a realization of the idea of fatigue. But the interest resides in the purely subjective nature of the trauma. In the case of Charcot's patient P, the 'shock' was unrelated to any fright or anticipated injury. P was out hunting and shot, as he thought, a fox. But to his horror the 'fox' proved to be a dog. His sense of guilt was intensified when the deceased was identified as his friend's dog! Later on the same day, while firing at a rabbit, P fell to the ground and, after a brief interval, lost consciousness. His right arm and leg were found to be paralyzed. Subsequently P lost his power of speech, although not the ability to write and read.

In P's case, a modern psychoanalyst could go far in 'reading' P's symptoms. His right arm was the 'guilty' one that fired the fatal shot, wronging both the dog and its master. P no doubt would 'rather have cut it off' to ensure it would never again commit such a crime. So he did the next best thing: the arm became limp and flaccid. Most likely P was 'speechless with horror,' literally as well as metaphorically as he stammered out his confession and apology, and in the sequel he became mute. Charcot in his lectures did not choose to go as far as this in the way of symbolic interpretation of symptoms. But in relation to a large class of cases he thought that a 'rudimentary paralysis' (we could say, a paralysis *in embryo*) is engendered by either an actual injury (which might be quite trivial), by an expectation of a specific injury (as in the case of Lys. or Janet's railway traveler), or by a shock to the emotions (as in the case of P or Justine 'Etch.'). 'One can understand that in a subject predisposed psychically, this rudimentary paralysis, provoked by the shock, becomes realized and developed to the full extent by reason of a mental elaboration, by a process of *auto-suggestion*.'[33]

The passage last quoted in one respect says rather more than the paragraphs given above which were taken from the *Dictionary* article of 1892. Charcot was particularly impressed by the lapse of time between the original trauma and the emergence of the hysterical symptom. In the examples quoted, a period of five to fifteen days is typical. Charcot thought of a suggestion related to the particular form of the trauma as being worked up by a process of *mental elaboration*. This phrase gave rise to many echoes. Breuer, in one of the papers collected in the epoch-making *Studies on Hysteria*, spoke of traumatic hysteria, consequent on a very frightening experience, in the following way:

> During the days following a railway accident, for instance, the subject will live through his frightful experiences again both in sleeping and waking, and always with the renewed affect of fright, till at last, after this period of 'psychical working out' [élaboration] (in Charcot's phrase) or of 'incubation,' conversion into a somatic phenomenon takes place.[34]

In the same collection of papers Freud speaks of Katharina, the innkeeper's daughter who consulted him while he was on vacation in the Hohe Tauern of Ost Tirol for mild hysterical symptoms consequent on 'moral shock,' as Charcot would have called it.

> Another peculiarity of Katharina's case, which, incidentally has long been familiar to us, is seen in the circumstance that the conversion, the production of hysterical phenomena, did not occur immediately after the trauma but after an interval of incubation. Charcot liked to describe this interval as the 'period of psychical working out' [élaboration].[35]

Readers familiar with Freud's *Interpretation of Dreams* will recall his term *secondary elaboration*, which refers to the transformation of the dream in the conscious memory after waking.

Freud and Breuer also found many other clues to the nature of hysteria in the observations reported at the Salpêtrière and in Charcot's remarks thereon. In somnambulistic or delirious phases of the hysterical attack the patient's *attitudes passion-elles*, could (as Charcot said) often be related to the emotions of the original trauma or sequence of traumas. Patients often adopted an attitude of alarm, or of defence against attack or injury by impact or crushing. Their hallucinations or utterances often referred directly to the traumatic experience, as with the patient Ler., whose convulsive deliria related to dogs, thieves, skeletons, and ghosts in direct correspondence to the series of traumas in her actual history; a rabid dog, a corpse, and robbery with violence. It was from the variety of case histories assembled by Charcot that Breuer was able to formulate the principle (much developed by Freud) that hysterical conversion (i.e., replacement of terror or anxiety by a physical symptom) could result either from a single very violent trauma or from accumulation of the effects of a series of traumas. Freud and Breuer found many such cases. Young Katharina developed her hysterical symptoms after a series of 'moral shocks' resulting from encounters with the innkeeper's sexual behavior. Breuer gave an example of hysteria in a young girl precipitated by fright when a cat jumped on her shoulder in the dark. But this physical trauma had been preceded by a series of 'moral shocks' —a sequence of attempted sexual assaults of varying degrees of brutality. A few days prior to the encounter with the cat, the girl had been attacked by a young man on the same dark staircase. Breuer went further still:

> In order for the repetition of an affect to bring about a conversion in this way, it is not always necessary that there should be a number of external provoking causes. The renewal of the affect in *memory* is often also enough if the recollection is repeated rapidly and frequently, immediately after the trauma and before its affect has become weakened.[36]

It was apropos of *élaboration* in another context, that Freud quotes a very striking phrase of Charcot's which I have not been able to find in his lectures but which Charcot may have used in the course of private discussion. Freud is speaking on his progress in the cure of his patient Frau Emmy von N.

On each occasion what was already present as a finished product in the unconscious was beginning to show through indistinctly. This idea, which emerged as a sudden notion, was worked over by the unsuspecting 'official consciousness' (to use Charcot's term) into a feeling of satisfaction, which swiftly and invariably turned out to be unjustified.[37]

Clearly, Charcot recognized grades or compartments of mental life, for so intelligent a man, speaking no matter how informally, could not conceivably have referred to an 'official' consciousness without realizing that this phrase by implication pointed to the existence of an 'unofficial' consciousness, even if only in a somewhat figurative sense.

Various observations would contribute to the notion that hysterics were capable of two psychic states separated by a kind of barrier. There was Charcot's *la belle indifférence des hystériques* exhibited by some of the patients, who behaved with a particular insouciance as if unconcerned by their symptoms and, indeed, as if unaware of them. There was also the range of ideas tinted with fear or emotion displayed by patients in the somnambulistic and delirious phases of their attacks, which vanished from memory on return to normal consciousness.

Breuer and Freud were much impressed by a phrase of Charcot's—*une condition seconde*; 'a second psychic state,' differing from normal consciousness. The phrase itself seems to have originated with Dr Azam, who studied the various psychic states of Félida X. It seems that Charcot imported the phrase from similar studies of 'multiple personality,' and applied it to states resultant on trauma. Charcot noted that Page in England, who had studied 'railway spine' and other traumatic hysterias, had emphasized the 'nervous shock' in accident cases in opposition to (physical) traumatic shock. The nervous shock was often combined with the physical shock, but could also be recognized as something distinct. In nervous shock, a peculiar mental condition sometimes developed. It was in this abnormal psychic state, thought Charcot, that autosuggestion produced the hysterical symptom, the patient's suggestibility being then exceptionally heightened. Charcot asked if this state was not closely related to the hypnotic state:

No doubt men are not in hypnotic sleep when they suffer falls or when later their paralyses come on. But is the nervous shock at and after the accident not equivalent (in predisposed subjects) to the cerebral condition which is determined in hysterics by hypnotism?[38]

Freud and Breuer postulated that stress could put a person into a *hypnoid state*: it was from emotions and suggestions received in the hypnoid state that the neurosis developed, but the ideas involved in the neurosis remained cut off from the official consciousness. It is interesting to see how closely related Freud's and Breuer's concept was to Charcot's, and it would be hard to deny Charcot the credit for having inspired it. The fact that Freud abandoned the idea in 1896 does not detract from its historical importance.

Charcot's *condition seconde* is in fact manifested in innumerable examples of stupors and twilight states in shock and fear syndromes.[39] Stupor can be occasioned merely by psychic trauma and moral shock. After the battle of Magenta, Napoleon III was for some hours reduced to a state of stupor—not by fear, but with horror at the many thousands of dead and dying. As regards twilight states, the hysteric sometimes experiences them and recapitulates features of the original trauma. The Charcot-Breuer-Freud thesis that 'shock' states can be assimilated into the deeper hypnotic states is one that finds powerful support today as indicated by Kretschmer:

Along with stupor in human fear psychosis and fear hysteria, we frequently find the twilight state, a hypnoid sleeplike or dreamlike state of consciousness which illustrates, without simultaneous motor paralysis, the death feint [found in animals] . . .; it affords protections against external physical and psychic forces and can culminate in true reactive somnolent states, or narcolepsy. As a reaction to fright and other emotional stimuli, the symptoms of both the cataleptic stupor and the hypnoid trance are closely related and frequently intermingled; similarly, there are also transitional and interpenetrating forms ranging from the mild to the pronounced twilight state and to the flurries of the hysterical attack, tremor neuroses, and the like. Finally . . . there is a pronounced tendency for experimental hypnosis to lead to hysterical twilight states; this obstructive tendency often appears in medical and lay hypnosis and betrays the inner relation between human hypnosis and the hysterical hypnoid.[40]

It is worth remarking in passing that fright or psychic shock can generate a condition displaying features akin to *la belle indifférence*. Survivors of the great earthquakes at Messina and Valparaiso comprised both some individuals who were plunged mute and motionless into stupors and others who showed a cheerfulness, quite incongruous in the circumstances, coupled with an apparent amnesia of the event and indifference to the horrors around them. For example, one man

. . . had lost his family in the earthquake and had narrowly escaped death himself. The tragedy seemed not to have made the slightest impression on him; he 'knew' nothing at all about it, although he saw his demolished home and heard his friends talk about it. He was seen *driving happily around in his automobile*; when anyone spoke to him, he became confused and laughed. Before that he had been a good husband and father. . . .[41]

Charcot refused to admit an essential distinction between traumatic neuroses resulting in hysterical conversion symptoms and hysterias not having a known traumatic origin. This insistence on the essential similarity of all conditions characterized by conversion symptoms was undoubtedly correct and is not negated by the recognition that we can distinguish between fear syndromes and the hysterical conversion that follows on some (though not all) of these states.[42]

Charcot has been taken to task for his belief that in addition to precipitating causes of hysteria, an innate predisposition to hysteria had to be postulated. There are various reasons why, rightly or wrongly, this supposition should have fallen (for a time at least) into disfavor. The idea of a 'hereditary taint' is always unpleasant. Hence, if the hereditary factors in hysteria were overstressed, a certain sense of shame was liable to attach to the invalid and his relatives. The other reason was Freud's eventual success in winning acceptance for his own discoveries. Freud found that episodes of family life played a great role in laying the basis for neurosis. Consequently, although he discussed the question of a predisposition to hysteria many times, he came in the end to lay greater stress on the environmental aspects; that is, the relations of the child with parents and siblings. But nonetheless, there were quite good reasons for Charcot and his contemporaries to hypothesize a hereditary basis for this class of ailments which, in Charcot's phrase, constituted a *famille neuropathique*. In the first place, during the very period when Pasteur and Koch were demonstrating the infective —and therefore environmental—component of so many diseases, Charcot and his fellow neuropathologists were manifesting the constitutional or inborn character of numerous neurological and other conditions. Many of these conditions, though absent in the young adult, come on in middle life and proceed with all the inevitability of a Greek tragedy, without showing any correlation at all with any discernable environmental feature. In other affections, some environmental factors could be ascertained to be of import, but nonetheless a residuum of constitutional susceptibility or predisposition seemed to remain. Charcot was by no means unaware of environmental factors. In his lectures on Senile and Chronic Diseases he shows a complete awareness of the work of Garrod and others on certain diseases. In a long discussion of gout, he comments on its strange regional and racial incidence. Thus in the nineteenth century, London had a notably high incidence of this disease, which oddly enough, said Charcot, seemed to strike groups as diverse as peers of the realm and Irish laborers engaged on large construction works. High living could hardly be blamed in the case of the laborers, Charcot said. There was a common factor, however: Some alcoholic beverages are more encouraging to gout than others, and the key to this fatality in the Irish building workers was the immense quantities of porter they consumed. Even nobler drinks carried their penalties. Charcot pronounced the dictum: 'There is gout in every glass of Burgundy or Hermitage.'[43]

Charcot and his predecessors such as Briquet, and some of his successors such as Janet and Babinski, were impressed by the number of hystericals encountered among their patients who had parents with hysteria, neuroses, or psychoses or who were epileptic. Thus Briquet claimed that 30 of every 100 of his patients had a parent with some type of mental disorder. Charcot quoted this figure in a lecture at which he presented a girl having sensory hemianesthesia, anesthesia of the left side, and a contracture of the left hand. Her mother had died from tuberculosis and her father in a lunatic asylum in Orleans; her brother was almost an idiot. When the child of a hysteric was hysterical, Charcot's contemporaries spoke of *similar heredity* (heredity of similitude); when the child was hysterical but the parent an epileptic or a psychotic, they spoke of *dissimilar heredity* (heredity by transformation).

Freud, too, in his early researches, was impressed by the fact that neurotics often had neurotic parents or siblings. But he saw that this fact admitted of distinct interpretations. It might correspond to a common inherited disposition; but it might signify only that neurotic behavior by one member of a family acts as an environmental cause of neurosis in another.[44] Freud therefore rightly criticized the familial evidence cited in support of the theory of hereditary transmission as lacking in cogency. Charcot's official pronouncements on the existence of a hereditary basis for hysteria were mild and infrequent, but according to Freud what he said privately was more emphatic, and tended to be elevated into a dogma by some of his pupils, namely, Guinon, Janet, and Gilles de la Tourette. On at least two occasions Freud cited Charcot's attitude to the etiology of tabes dorsalis and progressive muscular atrophy, to exemplify what in his own opinion was an excessive emphasis on inborn features of the patient's constitution.[45] Fournier and Erb had pointed to syphilitic infection as a powerful causative factor in some paralyses, a theory Charcot was in no haste to accept. Maybe Charcot was in error and Fournier and Erb were right. At this stage in history both views appear in retrospect to have been tenable by reasonable men.

Freud did not reject the possibility that innate constitutional factors play a part in hysteria. But he was much concerned to establish the importance of specific events (psychical and emotional) in the etiology of hysteria. And so, having made his strictures on Charcot and the latter's pupils, Freud puts forward the following moderate case, mildly expressed:

> Experience shows, as might have been anticipated, that among the problems of aetiology that of the quantitative relationship of the aetiological factors to one another should not be neglected. But one would not have guessed the fact which seems to follow from my observations, that heredity and the specific causes may replace one another quantitatively, that the same pathological effect will be produced by the co-existence of a very grave specific aetiology and a moderate degree of predisposition as by that of a severe neuropathic heredity with a slight specific factor. So that it is merely a quite possible extreme in this series when one finds cases of neurosis in which a tangible degree of hereditary predisposition is looked for in vain, provided that this deficiency is compensated for by a powerful specific factor.[46]

This somewhat abstract formulation may be readily understood if we proceed on the analogy of pulmonary tuberculosis. In the days when tuberculosis was rife in Western Europe (not so long ago, as a matter of fact), a tuberculous patient was very likely to have one or more tuberculous relatives. From this bare finding it might seem that the disease was primarily hereditary. There certainly is a strongly inherited constitutional factor in pulmonary tuberculosis. Each genetic constitution has its own individual degree of susceptibility, and very susceptible parents tend to have children who on average will be rather susceptible. But the character *susceptibility* does not occur in the population in two extreme grades only, low and high. Instead, it exists in every possible degree ranging from very high susceptibility to complete or almost complete immunity. Also, even high susceptibility is not of itself sufficient to condemn its possessor to 'consumption.' Infection and diet are very powerful causative agents. Poor nutrition, overcrowding, and bad housing kept tuberculosis active in Britain before World War II. Progress in housing, and medical services and adequate nutrition (since about 1930) have practically abolished new cases of the 'white scourge.'

It cannot be said that the question of hysterical predisposition to neurosis has yet been settled with any finality.[47] A study by Brown in 1942 on the relatives of neurotic patients suggested that there is a constitutional basis for some syndromes of the anxiety, hysterical, and obsessional types, and that there may be a factor common to all types of neurosis—namely, an anxious personality.[48] Slater, in 1943, investigated the relationships between personality traits and subsequent neuroses. He found that neurotic symptoms appeared as exaggerations of ordinary personality traits. Hysterical symptoms were correlated with hysterical traits of personality, though less strongly than obsessional neuroses and preexisting obsessional traits.[49] As to the personality traits themselves, one cannot assume blindly that these are entirely inborn, for that is to fall into the original *petitio principiae* of 'similar heredity.' One must assume that to some extent personality traits are malleable by the life history and familial situation. On the other hand, it would be unreasonable to postulate no constitutional or hereditary element whatever. Slater in 1944 propounded a 'heuristic theory of neurosis,' which is very much in accord with modern genetic ideas. The neurotically predisposed individual (like the person of high susceptibility to tuberculosis) is situated somewhere toward an extreme of normal human variation, having more than average susceptibility to environmental stresses, and this constitution is preponderantly determined by a very large number of genes of individually small effect.

The foregoing conclusion seems natural enough according to present-day ideas. One needs to recollect that the nineteenth century was almost totally devoid of any notions whatsoever concerning the mechanisms of inheritance. Weismann's theories met with little interest, and Galton's discoveries made little impact and, if anything, had a tendency to encourage the extreme hereditary view accompanied by neglect of environmental factors. As for Darwin, the burden of ignorance with which he valiantly struggled can hardly be appreciated until one has read Fisher's brilliant analysis of Darwin's thinking.[50] Mendel died still saying 'Mein Zeit wird kommen,' but his 'time' did not arrive until 1902. It should be recollected that Charcot *did* give weight to environmental factors. He spoke of hysteria as dependent on a special predisposition *and* on various exciting causes—*agents provocateurs*—that awakened hysteria where it lay latent in the predisposed individual. Although he said that 'some individuals seem to be hysterical from birth' (this with reference to cases of hysteria in young children), he said also that 'the greater number of those suffering from this affection are simply born susceptible to hysteria (*hystérisables*). . . .'[51] Any battles on this issue were, and are, largely battles about words. The whirligig of time brings in its changes, however, and certain classes of hysterics have been shown to be characterized not merely by particular personality traits, but by physical traits related to sexual underdevelopment and intersexual stigmata in their physical structure.[52]

Charcot was too loyal to the facts of observation to seek to prescribe any single physical or personality type as representing the hysterical predisposition. He was well aware of the so-called hysterical or histrionic personality noted in so many women patients. But he did not believe for a moment that hysterics were all of this type. Speaking of the melancholic condition of many of his male traumatized patients he observed:

This mental condition differs strangely from the brilliant and sparkling condition of mind which the exclusive study of hysteria in the female has accustomed us generally to consider as a speciality of those affected with this *grande névrose*.[53]

Charcot did not maintain that hysterics were in the main unintelligent people. Many of the patients he introduced to his class were, like Justine 'Etch.,' described as intelligent, or were comparable to the young Russian S, of whom Charcot said that he was imaginative, a reader of poetry, and a lover of music and books. Charcot would doubtless have agreed with Breuer, who wrote as follows in rebuttal of a view that he (Breuer) ascribed to Janet:

Every observer is largely under the influence of the subjects of his observation and we are inclined to believe that Janet's views were mainly formed in the study of the feeble-minded hysterical patients who are to be found in hospitals or institutions because they have not been able to hold their own in life on account of their illness.

In our opinion among hysterics may be found people of the clearest intellect, strongest will, greatest character and highest critical power. No amount of genuine, solid mental endowment is excluded by hysteria, though actual achievements are often made impossible by illness. After all the patron saint of hysteria, St Theresa, was a woman of genius with great practical capacity.

But on the other hand no degree of silliness, incompetence and weakness of will is a protection against hysteria. Even if we disregard what is a *result* of the illness, we must recognize the type of feeble-minded hysteric as a common one. Yet even so, what we find here is not torpid, phlegmatic stupidity but an excessive degree of mental mobility which leads to inefficiency.[54]

(To be fair to St Theresa, we ought to note that the department of human pathology over which she presides, as a help in time of trouble, is listed as 'Headaches.' Breuer was clearly of the same opinion as Sir Benjamin Brodie, that some four-fifths of pains in women were hysterical.)

Though Charcot believed that the ultimate or final cause of hysteria lay in the innate constitution of the patient, he was much more interested in the proximate or immediate causes of hysterical symptoms. In his search for a *causa efficiens*, he was much influenced by the numerous illustrations of the effect of the mind upon the body collected by Hack Tuke and published in 1872, and was guided more specifically by Professor Russell Reynolds' concept of *psychical paralyses* put forward in the British Medical Journal during 1869 (22). In Lecture XX, Charcot told his class :

Let us try to recognize at least in part the mechanism of the production of traumatic hysterical paralyses. . . . We must take a course apparently devious, and must return once more to a subject which has already occupied our attention. I mean those remarkable paralyses which have been designated *psychical paralyses, paralyses depending on ideas, paralyses by imagination*. Now, observe, I do not say *imaginary paralyses*, for indeed these motor paralyses of psychical origin are as objectively real as those depending on an organic lesion; they simulate them as you will soon see, by a number of identical clinical characters, which render their diagnosis very difficult.

Referring to Reynolds, Charcot continued :

It is well known that in certain circumstances an idea may produce a paralysis, and conversely that an idea may cause it to disappear; but between these two ultimate facts, many links appear obscure. Evidently this is a subject which would gain in clearness and precision if it could be submitted to experimental investigation.

Well, gentlemen, thanks to recent notions in relation to the science of hypnotic neurosis, it is possible to use experiment. In subjects in a state of hypnotic sleep it is possible to originate by the method of suggestion, or of intimation, an idea or coherent group of associated ideas, which *possess the individual,* and *remain isolated*, and manifest themselves by corresponding motor phenomena.

If the idea suggested be one of paralysis, real paralysis virtually ensues, and we see in such a case that it will frequently manifest itself as accentuated as that arising from a destructive lesion of cerebral substance.[55]

Researches on hypnotism in hysterical patients had proceeded at the Salpêtrière since 1878. Many controversies resulted, but they are not germane to the kind of demonstration of which Charcot is speaking, and which he gave annually in his professorial lectures from about 1882 onwards. Now, for reasons that will be considered later, the hysterical patients used as subjects for hypnosis at La Salpêtrière tended to enter one or the other of three somewhat different states of deep hypnosis. Charcot had christened these states *phases*, while making it clear that the three phases—*lethargy, catalepsy,* and *somnam-*

bulism were not necessarily encountered in that chronological order by the subject while going into deep hypnosis.

The state of *lethargy*, had all the appearance of profound slumber in which, as Charcot put it, 'mental inertia is so absolute that in general it is impossible to enter into relation with the hypnotized subject or to communicate any idea to him by any process.' But if the eyes of the lethargic subject were suddenly opened by the experimenter, the subject passed into the state of *catalepsy*. In catalepsy, the subject's limbs tended to retain any position imposed on them by the experimenter. 'In catalepsy,' said Charcot :

> certain phenomena of suggestion are easily obtained, and owing to their simplicity and their small tendency to become generalized, they are relatively easy of analysis. Here then, evidently, the study of hypnotic suggestion ought to commence. Here as in the preceding phase, there is mental inertia, but it is less profound, less absolute; it has become possible, indeed, to produce a sort of partial waking in the organ of the psychic faculties. Thus one can call into existence an idea, or a group of ideas connected together by previous associations. But this group set in action will remain strictly limited. There will be no propagation, no diffusion of the communicated movement; all the rest will remain asleep. Consequently the idea or group of ideas suggested, are met with in a state of isolation, free from the control of that large collection of personal ideas long accumulated and organized, which constitute the consciousness properly so called, the *ego*. It is for this reason that the movements which exteriorly represent the acts of unconscious cerebration are distinguished by their automatic and purely mechanical character. Then it is truly that we see before us the *human* machine in all its simplicity, dreamt of by de La Mettrie.[56]

For 1885, Charcot's language is remarkably advanced—indeed, modern. The 'coherent group of associated ideas,' which remains isolated and free from the consciousness or ego and only manifests itself in automatisms, is hardly to be distinguished from the unconscious *complex* of ideas occurring in psychoanalytical theory. (The word 'complex,' says Freud, became 'naturalized, so to speak, in psycho-analytic language,' having been introduced by the school of Jung around the year 1907.)[57]

It is fair to say that in the above passage quoted from Charcot, we have one of the earliest formulations of a theory of neurosis in terms of psychic contents maintaining themselves in isolation from the 'official consciousness.' Of course, he is speaking only of conditions artificially producible in hypnotized subjects, but the whole trend of the argument is directed toward showing that hysterical symptoms can be interpreted in terms of similar groups of associated 'ideas' cut off from consciousness. The final demonstration of this thesis was to be performed with somnambulic hypnotized patients. But prior to that, for the education of his class, Charcot—by way of entrée—carried out a subsidiary demonstration with a patient in a state of hypnotic catalepsy.

In this cataleptic condition, in the greater number of individuals, the only means by which we can enter into relation with the person hypnotised is through the *muscular sense*. The gesture alone, or the attitude in which we put the subject, suggests to him the idea which we wish to transmit to him. By shutting, for example, his fists in an aggressive attitude, you observe the head carried backwards, and the forehead, the eyebrows, and the root of the nose become corrugated with a menacing expression. Or, again, if you place the tips of his stretched-out fingers on his mouth, then the lips relax, he smiles, and all the face assumes an expression of softness totally opposed to what it just manifested.[58]

Whether on the basis of this demonstration Charcot was justified in saying that the operator has transmitted an idea to the subject is highly arguable. It would clearly be sufficient to say that by putting the fists in an aggressive attitude, a series of reflexes belonging to the primitive arousal system are called into action, and that the whole complex response is a pure automatism. Indeed, in a paper with Paul Richer, published in 1883 with the title 'Note on certain facts of Cerebral Automatism: Suggestion by the Muscular Sense,' Charcot rather implies this.[59] But there is a good deal to say on the two-way traffic between reflex-functioning on the one hand and conscious affects on the other. (Indeed, this is the whole issue at stake in debates on behaviorism.) If a man in a normal state of consciousness adopts an attitude of rage, then—inevitably, although in the best of tempers—he experiences subjectively some of the emotions of excitement and tension associated with actual anger or pugnacity, even though he does not feel the full affect of rage. Charcot would be very familiar with a *locus classicus* of this subject, the observations of Azam of Bordeaux, celebrated for the discovery of alternations of personality in 'Felida X.' Hypnotizing another young girl in the X household (in 1859), Azam found that,

> If during the period of catalepsy, I place the arms of Mlle X . . . in a position of prayer, and I let them stay for a certain time, she replies that she is only thinking of praying, and that she believes herself to be in church. If her head is inclined forward and arms bent, she feels her spirit invaded by a series of ideas of humility and contrition : the head high, she has feelings of pride.[60]

By way of clarification it should be said that catalepsy is a familiar feature of hypnosis, but that it is not always associated with unconsciousness. Cataleptic hypnosis as found at the Salpêtrière will be discussed later.

Charcot was very familiar with the system of reflexes governing the action of the facial muscles in producing physiognomic expression, for this had been elucidated by Duchenne de Boulogne. Duchenne's results were of great interest to Charcot and also to Darwin, who remarked that Duchenne's works in this field had been spoken lightly of, or quite passed over, by some of his countrymen. In 1872, Darwin published *The Expression of the Emotions in Man and Animals* as a footnote to *The Descent of Man*, and refers to Duchenne's *Mécanisme de la physionomie humaine* published in 1862. Darwin reproduced, with Duchenne's permission, many of the magnificent photographs illustrating movements of the facial muscles. Charcot therefore mentioned Duchenne's work to his class, in passing as it were, and then returned to the point he wished to emphasize in connection with the demonstration of attitudes induced in the cataleptic hypnotized subject :

> But the feature to which I specially wish to draw your attention at present is the way in which each impression thus originated by the intermediation of the muscular sense remains isolated without diffusion, and fixed, so to speak, during all the time that the muscular action maintains the members in the expressive attitude artificially produced.[61]

In other words, the cataleptic hypnotized person resembles the hysteric. An initial stimulus, for example, putting the hands into an aggressive attitude, activates a reflex system so that other muscles are drawn into the aggressive response. However, the stimulus does not need to be continuously reapplied. Once the aggressive *habitus* is established, it is maintained without erosion until a new stimulus is employed to cancel the original one. In the hysterical patient something very similar happens. As the result of stimuli, he develops a paralysis or a contracture, as did Dum. (mentioned in this chapter). Once established, the contracture persists without renewal of the original stimulus. It will be noted that at this stage of the argument Charcot does not speak of an idea, but uses a relatively noncommittal word, 'impression,' which could be thought of as a response or an 'unconscious idea.'

Charcot now speaks of another phase of hypnosis, the *somnambulistic*. To cut a long discussion short, it is only necessary to say that hypnotic somnambulism differed little, if at all, from the same state, obtainable with a certain proportion of subjects, recognized today in all textbooks on hypnosis and originally encountered by de Puységur about 1787. In Charcot's words,

> We have here to do solely with a state of obnubilation [of mind], mental torpor more or less accentuated. Here, again, without doubt, the awakening determined by suggestion remains partial, but the number of elements called into operation is less limited than in the preceding case, and frequently a diffusion occurs of the induced psychical phenomena sufficiently extensive to manifest a certain tendency to the reconstitution of the *ego*. Hence, it sometimes happens under these circumstances that the

injunction, the suggestion, becomes the occasion of a certain amount of resistance on the part of the subject. In all cases this yields to a little insistence. The movements in connection with the ideas suggested are consequently often very complex; they have not, therefore, that character of mechanical precision which they present in the preceding form : they assume the character of voluntary acts, more or less premeditated, even to the extent of leading one astray.

Further in the somnambulic stage all the senses are intact, and it may be said, indeed, that although the consciousness is in abeyance, the sensibility to communicated impressions is exalted. It consequently becomes easier to enter in relation by diverse means with the hypnotized person . . . suggestion can be effected by the aid of speech, either alone, or better, combined with gesture. . . . You will not be surprised to find that, in suggesting to a somnambulistic subject the idea of a morbid state, for example motor paralysis of the extremities, the paralysis becomes objectively manifest, and thus lends itself to our clinical investigation . . . that paralysis which we can make by the aid of suggestion, we are able at will to modify both in degree and character up to a point, and to unmake it equally well by suggestion. One can therefore anticipate that the study of paralysis thus artificially produced may one day be employed to elucidate the whole group of psychical paralysis.[62]

After this preamble, Charcot proceeded to introduce a hysterical girl, 'Greuz.,' who had a left hemianesthesia with full sensibility on the right side. Charcot remarked that she had been subjected to hypnotism on only four or five occasions,

so that in her case there is wanting the influence of training (*entrainement*) produced in subjects frequently hypnotized. Further I can assure you that the phenomena which you observe today are exactly the same as at our first experiment.

Greuz. was put into somnambulism. 'Your right hand is paralyzed,' said Charcot firmly. Greuz. demurred, saying Charcot was mistaken. But Charcot insisted in an accent of authority, and after a few minutes of this discussion, the hand hung flaccidly.

All active movement of the arm was abolished, as well as all resistance to passive movements. Very interestingly, the hand, the arm, the shoulder, and part of the chest—previously normal—now showed complete anesthesia. The genuineness of the anesthesia was verified by demonstrating to the class that violent torsion of the joints produced no sign of feeling, and that no pain or sensation was evidenced in Gruez.'s face on faradizing the nerve trunks of the arm even to the extent of causing violent contraction of the muscles. Charcot now pointed out to the class, with a certain air of justifiable satisfaction, that the symptoms produced artificially under hypnosis in Greuz. were in almost all respects identical with those occurring as hysterical symptoms in the previously mentioned patients Pin. and Porcz.

In the next lecture of the series of 1885, Charcot went further. By suggestion he produced the paralysis and corresponding anesthesia in Greuz. piecemeal. He first suggested immobility of the shoulder joint, which ensued, Greuz. however, being able to move elbow, wrist, and fingers quite freely. Pricking the shoulder, chest, and upper arm with a pin Charcot mapped out the anesthetic area. It extended somewhat over the right-hand part of the collarbone region and down the arm to a level about two inches above the elbow. Its boundary was a sharply defined arc, just as in anesthesias of hysterical origin. Charcot next induced paralysis of the elbow and showed that the resulting anesthesia extended down the forearm, to a level about two inches above the wrist. Finally he paralyzed the wrist. Only the fingers retained voluntary mobility. Anesthesia was bounded by a line passing diagonally across the hand from the base of the thumb to the base of the little finger. Greuz.'s 'symptoms' were now almost identical, even to the detailed boundaries of the anesthetic zone, with those of Porcz. Charcot now applied the *coup de grâce* and paralyzed Greuz.'s fingers with accompanying anesthesia. Her 'symptoms' were now those of Pin.

Charcot now unmade Greuz.'s symptoms, proceeding by segments upward from the hand and verifying at each stage the corresponding retreat of the anesthesia. To show that Greuz. was not an exceptional case, Charcot repeated the entire demonstration with a second patient, 'Mesl.' Lastly he told the class that in some cases he had been able to implant the suggestion of paralysis without anesthesia, suggesting to the subject that move-ment alone would be lost and that sensibility would remain intact. This was distinctly more difficult to achieve, he intimated, than paralysis with associated anesthesia.

Charcot carried out similar demonstrations year after year in his official lectures and similar ones in the informal Tuesday lectures. Since Freud was at the Salpêtrière from the autumn of 1885 to the summer of 1886, it is likely that he saw the demon-strations done with the self-same patients—Pin., Porcz., Greuz., and Mesl. Freud's earliest theory of hysteria relates very closely to a remark made by Charcot at the end of this demonstration :

> No doubt the men [i.e., Pin. and Porcz.] were not in a hypnotic sleep when they had their falls or when later their paralysis came on. But in this respect it may be enquired whether the mental condition occasioned by the emotion, by the nervous shock experienced at the moment of the accident and for some time after, is not equivalent in a certain measure, in subjects predisposed as Porcz. and Pin. were, to the cerebral condition which is determined in 'hysterics' by hypnotism . . . because of the annihilation of the *ego* produced by the hypnotism in the one case, and, as one may suppose, by the nervous shock in the other, that idea once installed in the brain takes sole possession and acquires sufficient domination to realise itself objectively in the form of paralysis. . . .
>
> I give you, gentlemen, that explanation for what it is worth, and without attaching to it more importance than it merits.[63]

As we recall, Breuer and Freud took up the idea that the foundation for a hysterical symptom was laid when the patient, on account of stress and strain or as a result of physical or psychic trauma, was in the *condition seconde* or hypnoid state, and that this foundation was then elaborated by a process of *autosuggestion*, with a cutting off or isolation of the symptom from the consciousness or ego.[64] Hence we can hardly deny to Charcot a formative role in the foundation of psychoanalysis and the modern discovery of the unconscious.

Another favorite demonstration by Charcot concerned the artificial production of mutism. He presented two cases of artificially induced mutism in hysterical women patients who, prior to the experiment to which they were being submitted, had never been in communication with hysterical mutes, although they had been in daily contact with patients afflicted with labio-glosso-laryngeal paralysis.

These women are unable to cry out, to articulate a single word, or even to whisper; and yet the general movements of the tongue and lips are quite free from any affection; they continue to be able to express themselves by writing and by gesture, and their intelligence is quite unaffected.

I bring them before you now, awake, but still mute; I ought to tell you how the phenomenon of mutism may be artificially produced. The patient being plunged into the somnambulic stage of hypnotism, you commence by conversing with her for a few minutes, then gradually you approach closer and closer to her, and finally pretend neither to hear nor understand her . . . you continue to practice the same ruse . . . the voice of the subject becomes progressively lower, and in the last stage *aphonia* becomes complete and there is an impossibility of articulation.

Artificial mutism, obtained during the somnambulic period, persists as you see in the waking state. I dare not allow this experiment to be prolonged too much, for I have remarked on many occasions that hysterical symptoms artificially produced during hypnotism are more difficult to be made to disappear in a waking stage in proportion as they are allowed to persist for a longer time.

This lecture is annotated (probably by Pierre Marie) to say that one of the women seemed to be vividly impressed by all that was said. The following morning, shortly after waking, she suddenly regained her speech.

At the end of the demonstration Charcot said :

Gentlemen, the possibility of giving rise to the syndrome *hysterical mutism* artificially by means of suggestion, appears to us to indicate sufficiently clearly the point of departure of all the phenomena; and one is thus able to suppose the mechanism of its development. It is in the grey cortex of the cerebral hemisphere that we must seek for the dynamical lesion whence emanate the symptoms in question; and the mechanism that is to be invoked in such conditions is none other than that which acts in the production of psychical, or, if you like it better, mental paralysis.[65]

Some later writers, no doubt misled by quoting at second hand, having (as Guillain says) not read Charcot's lectures, tend to use the reference to 'dynamic' lesion against him, as if he had said 'structural' lesion. But clearly, though we cannot acquit Charcot of having expressed himself discreetly, we cannot ignore his broad hint that events in the brain were best thought of, in this connection, in a very broad sense and were not to be distinguished easily from psychic or ideational events.

At the time of his death in 1893, Charcot had not drawn together into a single fabric the various ideas on hysteria which he had put out from time to time. Working entirely from the facts of observation as determined by himself and his predecessors, he had merely offered a series of suggestions, working hypotheses, and broad hints, without seeking to draw them together into a synthesis. But according to his pupil, Professor Joffroy, when 'death surprised him,' Charcot was in the process of generalizing his findings (i.e., the effect of psychogenic factors, the period of 'elaboration,' and the patient's creation of his illness by a sort of autosuggestion) and 'developing a theory of the psychological origin of all hysteric manifestations.' A few days before his death, Charcot told Georges Guinon that 'his [Charcot's] concept of hysteria had become decadent and his exposition of the pathology of the nervous system must be revised.'[66] We can only speculate on the form Charcot's synthesis would have taken. What role would he have ascribed to 'reflex hyperexcitability'? Would there have been an 'unconscious' in Charcot's system? And so on. Would depth psychology have taken a somewhat different route of development? Would the study of the unconscious have met with less resistance if launched with all the authority of *Le Professeur de La Salpêtrière*?

But Charcot had done enough to give Freud a springboard for diving into the unconscious. Here is Freud's testimony:

What impressed me most of all while I was with Charcot were his latest investigations on hysteria, some of which were carried out under my own eyes. He had proved, for instance, the genuiness of hysterical phenomena and their conformity to laws (*introite et hic dii sunt*), the frequent occurrence of hysteria in men, the production of hysterical paralyses and contractures by hypnotic suggestion and the fact that such artificial products showed, down to their smallest details, the same features as spontaneous attacks which were often brought on traumatically. Many of Charcot's demonstrations began by provoking in me and in other visitors a sense of astonishment and an inclination to sceptism, which we tried to justify by an appeal to one of the theories of the day. He was always friendly and patient in dealing with such doubts, but he was also most decided; it was in one of these discussions that (speaking of theory) he remarked, '*la n'empêche pas d'exister*' [you can't stop things from existing], a *mot* which left an indelible mark upon my mind.[67]

Freud also wrote in his obituary of Charcot:

At one point Charcot's work rose above the level of his general treatment of hysteria and took a step which gives him for all time the glory of being the first to elucidate hysteria. While he was occupied with the study of hysterical paralyses appearing after traumas, the idea occurred to him to reproduce by artificial means such paralyses as he had previously carefully differentiated from organic disturbances; for this purpose he took hysterical patients and placed them in a state of somnambulism by hypnotism. He succeeded in producing a faultless demonstration and proved thereby that these paralyses were the result of specific ideas holding sway in the brain of the patient at moments of special disposition. With this the mechanism of an hysterical phenomenon was for the first time disclosed, and on this incomparably fine piece of clinical research his own pupil Janet, and also Breuer and others, based their theories of the neurosis which, while agreeing with the medieval view, replaces the 'demon' of priestly imagination by a psychological formula.[68]

CHAPTER V

Cure, Faith, and Healing

THE SUBJECTIVE element in conversion hysteria is evidenced not only by the sudden onset of symptoms, but equally by the fact that on occasion normal function restores itself in an equally abrupt way. The *locus classicus* is Herodotus' story of Croesus' son, a deaf-mute who, seeing a Persian soldier about to kill his father, burst into speech; which is a counterpart to the myth of Iphiclus, who developed a traumatic neurosis occasioned by seeing his father coming toward him with a blood-stained knife.[1] Many instances of sudden relief were observed at the Salpêtrière and noted by Charcot in his lectures. Symptoms quite often disappeared after a hysterical attack. Charcot devoted a whole lecture to the case of Le Log., the patient who (it will be recalled) developed paralysis of the legs after an accident in which he believed—erroneously—that a cart had passed over his legs. As for Pin., Charcot cured the paralysis of his right arm by finding a hysterogenic point. Pressure precipitated Pin.'s first hysterical attack. Subsequently the arm had full motility. Charcot remarks that the arm had taken no part in the attack. Observations of this kind, reported by Charcot, explain Janet's remark (something of an exaggeration) to the effect that Charcot had noted that it was beneficial for certain patients to have convulsive crises, and that Charcot even went so far as to advise that in such cases a crisis should be induced.[2]

Apropos of Le Log.'s spontaneous cure, Charcot tells us that it was consequent upon a convulsive seizure of great severity in which his feet struck the bar at the end of the bed with so much force that it became displaced. Whereupon the attack terminated; the patient rose from the bed and commenced to walk, weakly at first but with normal strength after a few hours.[3] In this case an important role may have been played by the shock transmitted to the paralyzed legs on account of the feet striking the bed. At the Salpêtrière they often had success in relieving a hysterical paralysis by electrical stimulation of the muscles in question. One famous demonstration concerned a girl of nineteen, a laundress who followed her calling on a boat on the Seine, who had developed traumatic hysteria with paralysis of hand, arm, and right shoulder subsequent to a shelf carrying heavy objects falling on her head while she slept. In the lecture hall Charcot proceeded to faradize the shoulder and arm muscles. Pierre Marie says in a foot-note :

> At the end of a minute the sensibility had entirely returned to this region, without transfer [i.e., to the left shoulder as in the phenomenon of *transfert*]. A minute later the sensibility had returned throughout the entire limb and the paralysis had gone. The patient was then able to use the arm as well as ever, and went round among the audience vigorously shaking them by the hand, desirous of proving how real was the recovery they had just witnessed.[4]

But physical shocks were not necessary or generally effective in producing spontaneous cure. Charcot narrated some interesting examples among his patients of cure resulting from 'moral shock.' One woman had as her only symptom a contracture of the lower right leg which persisted for two years, until it vanished suddenly one day when she was accused of theft. Another patient recovered suddenly from a contracture of the right side of eighteen months' duration on experiencing an unexpected disappointment. Of another patient with a long-persisting contracture of the leg Charcot said :

> On account of the misconduct of this patient, I was obliged to give her a strong admonition and declare I should turn her out of the hospital. Next day, the contracture had entirely disappeared. This fact is all the more important because her convulsive attacks [had long ceased]. For two or three years the contracture was the only manifestation of the 'great neurosis.' . . .[5]

In a footnote to the famous lecture in which the symptoms of Pin. and Porcz. were reproduced in Greuz., Charcot considered the method of 'injunction' :

> We know that a sudden injunction sometimes determines the cure of a psychical paralysis of long standing, which may have resisted the most varied therapeutic agencies. Thus, for example, a patient is forcibly made to leave her bed, in which she may have long remained motionless from a paraplegia of this kind; and being placed on her feet, she is told to 'walk', and forthwith she walks. Here we have an example of a 'miraculous' cure which explains many others. There is nothing better established than these facts, to which I have frequently borne testimony.
>
> Nevertheless, we cannot be too guarded, even with the best intentions, against assuming the part of a miracle-worker, for even in a case of psychical paralysis of an undoubted nature injunction is a remedy, the mechanism of which we know little. Failure would compromise the authority of the operator, and subject him to ridicule. . . . To proceed by a slow and progressive method of mental training will always be more prudent, and often more efficacious.[6]

Charcot was not concerned for the dignity *per se* of the physician, but only in so far as it was necessary to retain the patient's confidence in his doctor, because a certain degree of authority was indispensable if the 'mental training' were to have any chance of success. In one of his Tuesday lectures he expressed himself more animatedly :

> A miracle-monger can say to his patient 'Get up and walk.' Why should we not play the thaumaturge, since it is for the good of our patients? Well, gentlemen, I do not say categorically that you should never do anything of the kind. In certain cases, if you are quite sure of your diagnosis, perhaps you will do well to take the risk. You had better walk cautiously in such matters. Do not forget that, in practice, you have to deal with questions of taste, opportunity, and, let me add, medical dignity, for the importance of this last must never be overlooked. Do not forget that nothing can make you seem more absurd than to predict

with great pomp and circumstance a result which will perhaps never be achieved.

Suggestion is a difficult agent to handle; it is, if you will permit the metaphor, a drug whose accurate dosage is far from easy. The English, who are a preeminently practical people, have a saying, 'Don't prophesy unless you know.' I am in full agreement with their outlook upon this point, and I advise you to guide your own actions by so excellent a precept.[7]

Charcot would be quite familiar with a famous anecdote of the Paris hospitals quoted by the *American Journal of Insanity* in 1865, and also by Hack Tuke. In 1849 a little girl, Louise Parguin, 'whom excessive fear had rendered dumb, and paralytic in all her limbs,' was brought to the Hôtel-Dieu.

> For two months everything had been done by the physicians but to no purpose. In despair her father came with his child to Paris. The girl, who had heard of the great city, its great physicians and the Hôtel-Dieu spoken of in the most extravagant way, arrived full of faith to be cured. In the evening I saw her dumb and paralytic; and, displeased at finding such a patient in the hospital made no prescription. She was in the same state the next morning; I put off all treatment. During the day she began to speak, the day after to move her limbs, and on the third day she walked about the wards completely cured. Her faith had saved her.[8]

But Charcot was aware that few patients were impressionably so preconditioned as this. Even La Salpêtrière could not compete with Lourdes in the matter of faith, nor Dr Charcot with St Louis or 'Monsieur de Paris' (Deacon François de Pâris).

In his official lectures Charcot hardly ever referred directly to hypnotic therapy—the method which, by fits and starts, had been coming into vogue since about 1860. Possible reasons for this reticence will be considered later. Hypnosis offers certain advantages. Cure by injunction promises more chance of success than do commands to the patient in the waking state. Also the physician's prestige with the patient is perhaps placed less in jeopardy. Hypnotic therapy was certainly being attempted in the

Salpêtrière during the 1880's, at least experimentally if not routinely. This emerges from a remark of Charcot which also suggests that the Salpêtrians had a certain amount of success with the method. Charcot concluded the great Lecture XXII by outlining the methods employed in treatment of Pin. and Porcz., which he used to exemplify the general Salpêtrière approach to cure of hystericals. 'The treatment consists of two elements. On the one hand, it is in a sense indirect, in that it relates either to the general state or to the hysterical diathesis.'[9]

This general treatment consisted of cold showers or sulphur baths given several times a week, and applications of static electricity on alternate days. Their experience, said Charcot, was that these procedures did tend to restore sensibility, that is, they diminished anesthesias, and mitigated hysterical attacks and other symptoms.

But Charcot wished especially to emphasize the second part of the treatment, based on the idea that hysterical paralysis is caused by a mechanism analogous to the production of paralyses by suggestion under hypnosis. Somewhat significantly he refers to 'The various attempts at hypnotization which we made in these two men, and which, if they had succeeded, would have singularly lightened our task.'[10] Clearly, therefore, Charcot had no hostility to the employment of hypnotic injunction for the relief of symptoms, and the method was in use in some degree at the hospital. His statement also implies that they had found it efficacious. Equally clearly its utility was zero if the patient could not be hypnotized. After this somewhat indirect reference, Charcot proceeds to the message he particularly wished to convey to the medical students and young physicians—the *need for acting psychically by persuasion* :

In the first place we acted, and continue to act every day on their minds as much as possible, affirming in a positive manner, a fact of which we are ourselves perfectly convinced—that their paralysis, in spite of its long duration, is not incurable, and that, on the contrary, it will certainly be cured by means of appropriate treatment, at the end possibly of some weeks, if they would only be good enough to aid us.[11]

Charcot's exposition indicates three distinct elements. One was the use of suggestion, what Janet has called 'the appeal to the patient's automatism.'[12] This is reinforced by invoking an emotional force, loyalty to the physician as implied by the phrase, 'if they would only be good enough to aid us.' Lastly, Charcot implies an appeal to the voluntary intention of the patient.

Later writers have discussed the hysteric in terms of a division of the 'will,' or in terms of the diminution of normally orientated conation, so that the patient is dominated by drives tending to perpetuate his symptoms. Kretschmer in our own day describes the hysteric as having two opposite drives : the will to get well and lead a fully functional life, and the will to persist in being an invalid.[13] Whether this second 'will' can properly be so called is another matter, but it is certainly a useful shorthand and compact figure of speech. Janet noted the *abulia* of hystericals, that is, the lack of normal functional willpower, thus putting emphasis not so much on the will to invalidism as upon the feebleness of the normal life-drive.[14] Charcot's prescription was, in any event, directed at buttressing the patient's normal instinct to return to a full life. Janet felicitously applied the term 're-education' to Charcot's program for his patients.

Charcot outlined a second feature of the course of re-education :

> . . . the affected members were submitted to methodical exercise. We availed ourselves of the voluntary movements which still subsisted, though in a feeble degree, in the two patients, and we tried to progressively augment the energy of these by a very simple method. A dynamometer was placed in the hand of each of them, and they were exhorted to squeeze it with all their power, and to progressively increase the reading.[15]

Reeducation as a concept in therapy goes back to Claudius Chervin, the pioneer of training deaf-mutes, who proposed that to treat stammering, the attention and the conscious will of the sufferers must be concentrated on the actual processes of breathing and speech formation during a course of special exercises.[16] But Janet says that it was Charcot who developed the first interesting systematization of methods of reeducation.[17] Since these patients had no lesions of the nervous system, reeducation was possible, at least in principle. Charcot notably demonstrated that, for the treatment to be a success, the subject's attention must be concentrated upon the movement he was to perform and upon the sensations of this movement. Charcot was therefore able to say with justice that in the imposed physical exercises, no less than with direct persuasion, 'we act psychically.' If the patient had no voluntary movement in the paralyzed limb, the doctor himself moved it while the patient concentrated attention on what was being done, watching the movement and noting the sensations. The patient then had to describe the action and sensations in words and had to reproduce it voluntarily with the corresponding unaffected limb. Patients frequently recovered some slight motion in the paralyzed member, and then could exercise regularly with the dynamometer. Charcot would also attach an indicator to the end of a paralyzed finger so that the patient could better appreciate its movements. The method had considerable successes, as reported by Charcot's pupils Paul Richer, Gilles de la Tourette, Seglas, Féré, and Lagrange.[18]

In Charcot's clinic Chervin's method was applied systematically to hysterical mutism, the patient being required to touch the doctor's chest and larynx to acquaint himself with the movements and vibrations. First he learned by degrees to make voluntary changes in respiration, then to make sounds, and finally to practice the repetition of syllables and words. Analogous systems of reeducation were employed at the Salpêtrière and elsewhere for treatment of astasia and abasia and contractures, as well as for choreas and tics. Charcot and Guinon were somewhat reserved about the prospect of cure of tics, but Brissaud and Henri Meige of Charcot's circle refined various methods of reeducation. Without doubt the Salpêtrière gave considerable impetus to methods of reeducation, which came to be applied to organic paralyses by Leyden and Frenkel. Frenkel's methods were introduced into the Salpêtrière by Professor Raymond, Charcot's successor, so that a wheel had turned full cycle and Charcot's studies in hysteria eventually benefited a later generation of neurological patients. Pitres, a pupil of Charcot's who became professor at Bordeaux, applied similar methods to habit-spasms such as tics and developed an approach based on concentration and control of breathing. Charcot himself seems not to have attempted reeducation in the cure of occupational cramps such as writer's cramp, for which he advised prolonged abstention from writing.

In explaining the method of reeducation with reference to Porcz. and Pin., Charcot hazarded a few words by way of theory:

> Here we act *psychically*. It is well known . . . that the production of an image, or of a mental representation, no matter how summary or rudimentary it may be of the movement to be executed, is an indispensable preliminary condition to the execution of that movement. But it is probable that, in the case of our two male patients, the conditions which normally preside over the representation of the mental image have been so seriously affected as to render its formation impossible, or at least very difficult, in consequence of an inhibitory action exercised over the cortical motor centres by the fixed idea of motor weakness. It is to that circumstance that the objective realization of the paralysis is principally due.[19]

He gave a battery of references to psychological writers of the day to support the thesis that the execution of a movement requires the presence of an image of that movement in the mind. On this line of argument a paralysis is explained in terms of an idea of muscular weakness which inhibits the formation of the idea of making an arm movement. Charcot thought of the exercises done very consciously by the patient as strengthening the idea of movement. He used a somewhat neurological terminology when he said that exercise tended 'to revive in the [motor] centres the motor representation, which is a necessary preliminary to the voluntary movement,'[20] but it is clear that he believed that a formulation primarily in terms of mental events, and in psychological language, was more appropriate to an understanding of the problem than a more mechanistic hypothesis.

Féré, studying twenty-three cases of hysterical paralysis which had yielded successfully to reeducation, gave an explanation that echoed Charcot's remark concerning the motor centers and played down the psychological formulation. Of this explanation Janet says:

> He considered that the beneficial results were to be explained by the stimulation of the brain centres corresponding to the paralysed regions. This phraseology, half psychological and half anatomical, conveyed no precise significance, and was indeed somewhat absurd; still it presented an image which had its uses for the moment, since it enabled doctors to understand the psychological facts which they had to translate into their customary speech. Féré's phrase has been used a good deal.[21]

We can suspect that many of the 'explanations' given by Charcot to his professional audiences which so often appeared to be facing both ways—part psychological and part in terms of the cerebral cortex—were not given in this hybrid form to enable him to hedge his bets, but to present images that would have their uses for the moment and assist the education of doctors in the psychological approach to the causes and cure of the neuroses.

While still on the subject of Pin. and Porcz., Charcot added a couple of interesting practical remarks. Considerable progress was made with their paralyses and the return of sensation to the affected arms, but there was no concomitant improvement of their other hysterical stigmata, nor remission of their hysterical attacks. In the case of Porcz., his recovery from paralysis was unstable, for in February 1886 he relapsed after quarreling with another patient over a game of draughts, the emotion bringing the paralysis on again.

In subsequent lectures Charcot discussed a case of traumatic hysterical 'hip disease' and another method of treatment of paralyses and contractures. 'We must never let hysterical contracture drag on,' he said, and treatment ought to start as soon as possible after onset by massaging the muscles. It was often found that the contracture was ameliorated at least temporarily, if only in the sense of being reduced to a flaccid paralysis. In this condition, reeducation could be embarked upon. Why was massage effective? Gilles de la Tourette, Charcot's assistant especially interested in curative techniques, said merely that it acted 'in virtue of a mechanism which we do not understand.'[22] Féré referred it to stimulation of the cortical centers.[23] Charcot in the relevant lecture said that massage was effective because of the hysterical nature of the subject. 'One might say the massage represents a sort of local hypnotism.' (i.e., massage works by suggestion.)

Gilles de la Tourette filled the three thick volumes of his *Traité clinique et thérapeutique de l'Hystérie d'après l'enseignement de la Salpêtrière* with case histories and attempted methods of cure. With many patients progress was slight and partial, with amelioration of a few symptoms only. These were the chronic cases often resulting from severe trauma, and sometimes long established before Charcot and coworkers received them. But, on the basis of his experience, Charcot spoke optimistically of the chances of cure with young patients, specially if correct treatment was instituted promptly:

> . . . one can very frequently manage to quench an attack of nascent, or infantile hysteria at its outset, especially in the male. [But] when this neurosis has become inveterate and occurs in adults, the chances of success though still great, are much more problematical.[24]

Charcot told his class several interesting case histories of juvenile hysteria. He saw a boy of thirteen years in consultation with 'a very distinguished physician, who displayed the greatest scepticism about hysteria in general and particularly concerning hysteria in childhood.' Charcot stopped the major hysterical attacks by pressures on hysterogenic points and prescribed tonics and hydrotherapy. Most important, he prescribed *isolation*, 'so as to withdraw him from the influence of his parents who petted him too much.' The boy was cured in three months.[25]

Another boy, aged thirteen, was hard working, bright and intelligent with healthy parents. For several months he had intense headaches. The physicians at his home in the south of Russia gave a very unfavorable prognosis, doubtless assuming a brain tumor. The boy's father (described as very impressionable and nervous, but otherwise normal), loving his son to distraction, undertook the voyage to Paris.

From the very first interview, we were able to give him hope. Not only will the child live, but we can affirm without hesitation that the child will make a complete recovery. The headache was in the habit of returning every evening about 5 p.m. followed shortly afterwards by convulsive attacks. The occurrence of the attack at the same time of day for five months, offers a strong presumption of hysteria.[26]

The diagnosis was confirmed by finding right hemianesthesia, with diminution of taste, smell, hearing, and color perception on the right-hand side.

It is interesting to note the deportment of the father at the expected time of attack. He takes out his watch and questions his son and asks if he is suffering. If the reply is 'Yes' he displays an amount of solicitude which is respectable, no doubt, but which certainly tends to foster the patient's condition and to maintain the regularity of his symptoms.[27]

Consequently, in addition to the customary tonics, static electricity, and hydrotherapy, Charcot prescribed isolation, essentially from the father, 'so as to withdraw him [the boy] from the parental solicitude, which serves only to perpetuate the excitable nervous condition; or at least I shall enjoin a firmer and less sympathetic behaviour on the part of the father.'[28]

The father, as it happened, would not consent to be separated, and every day at the same hour he awaited the attack, behavior that never failed to produce it in the same manner as before. The boy was then placed in a sanatorium, but the father prowled around outside all day earnestly questioning anyone who emerged from the building as to his son's condition. Eventually Charcot persuaded the father to allow real isolation, and the cure was completed within a month.

The theme of *expectation* and fixed ideas of *inevitability* as productive of attacks by suggestive force was touched on again by Charcot when introducing two lectures (XVI and XVII) entitled 'Spiritualism and Hysteria' and 'Isolation in the Treatment of Hysteria.' He referred to Françoise Fontaine, *La possédée de Louviers*, whose adventures were recounted in a sixteenth-century document reprinted in 1883 in the *Bibliothèque Diabolique*.[29] Charcot said that prior to the 'possession,' her imagination had been held in a constant state of tension by the wicked spirit which 'returned' each night to the house where she lived. But on this occasion he was more concerned to stress the importance of certain types of febrile excitement in the etiology of hysteria. 'Gentlemen,' he said,

> It is undoubtedly true that whatever forcibly strikes the mind, whatever strongly impresses the imagination, is singularly favourable, in subjects predisposed, to the development of hysteria . . . perhaps nothing is more efficacious . . . than the belief in the marvellous and the supernatural which is fostered and exaggerated by excessive religious practices, and the related order of ideas, spiritualism and its practices.[30]

Charcot would have in mind the *convulsionnaires* of Saint Médard, as well as similar convulsionarics who were among the patients treated by Mesmer in Paris and later by the Abbé Faria. Scenes of religious enthusiasm were familiar not only in the Latin countries but among the new sects proliferating in America and were characterized by an excessive emotionalism reminiscent of the original Shaker immigrants from England who may have derived in part from the fanatical Camisards or 'French Prophets.' Nowadays, Spiritualism seems a quiet and sedate pursuit, but we need to remember that during the latter half of the nineteenth century it enjoyed great vogue in America, Britain, and some European countries as a form of recreation and excitement, being practiced by numerous families and groups with no special mediumistic talent or understanding, purely as an escape from the boredom of the narrow and circumscribed existence pertaining to the middle station in life.

Charcot told of a case where dabbling in the forms of spiritualism, done ignorantly and unreflectively, had precipitated a familial epidemic of *grande hystérie*. Sublieutenant X was an officer in a military prison. 'Life in penitentiary cannot be very gay,' observed Charcot. Indeed, X and his family lived in dark and cramped rooms, looking out only into the prison courtyard. Life being terribly monotonous, the officers' wives earnestly conducted spiritualist séances daily for a year. On Fridays Lieutenant X also took part in table-turning. During the school holidays, on account of a message that 'Julie will be the medium,' their daughter aged thirteen took part in an all-day séance and went into trance from which her father aroused her by throwing water in her face. However, a neighbor then took her away for an evening séance. Julie produced automatic writing in an uncharacteristic handwriting. The hand with which she had written the message went into convulsive tremor, and Julie passed into a hysterical attack with delirium and great movements (clownism). Her attacks continued for three months and communicated themselves to her brother François aged eleven and in lesser degree to her brother Jacques aged twelve, who developed a tic with facial spasms and had delirious phases. Whenever the children encountered one another in the house, Julie would have an attack and the boys would follow suit.

Charcot quoted this case as exemplifying both the hysterogenic tendency of 'constant tension of mind,' and appropriate methods of treatment. The children were admitted to the Salpêtrière in order to effect their removal from the place of onset of their malady and separation from one another and from the parents whose presence would have nullified all treatment. Julie was placed in a female ward of the *Clinique* (which was for temporary, not chronic neurotics), and the boys were put in the only men's ward then possessed by the *Clinique*. Separation was thus achieved, even though to an imperfect degree. The parents engaged not to visit without Charcot's express permission. On the physical side, the children were given tonics and treatment with static electricity. But Charcot placed chief reliance 'on Isolation; i.e., moral treatment' because, 'the psychic element plays a very important part in most of the cases of this malady.' He regretted the fact that complete isolation from cases of convulsive hysteria was not possible at that time in public hospitals, but they had to do the best they could. As regards to management,

The patients are placed under the direction of competent and experienced persons. They are generally religious people who by long practice have become very expert in the management of this sort of patient. A kind but firm hand, a calm demeanour, and much patience, are here indispensable conditions.[31]

(The nursing staff of the Salpêtrière consisted, subsequent to Florence Nightingale and the Crimean War, of some secular nurses such as Mlle Bottard, Chief Nurse in the *Service du Professeur Charcot*, and also of numerous lay sisters, dressed as nuns, though not under vows, who had dedicated themselves to the voluntary care of the poor. Originally, in the days of St Vincent de Paul, these were under a sister superior and twenty-six sister officers.) Charcot continues:

The parents are systematically excluded up to the time that a notable amelioration occurs; and then the patients are allowed, as *a sort of recompense*, to see them; at first at long intervals, and then more and more frequently in proportion as the improvement becomes more obvious.

Hysteria recently acquired, especially in young subjects and particularly in males, could often be stifled at the outset if it were possible to persuade the parents to undertake energetic measures at the beginning, and not to wait until the disease has taken deep root and become developed from having been a long time abandoned to itself.[32]

Six weeks later Charcot made good his words by presenting the three children substantially cured. He said: 'There is every reason to hope that this little family drama, or as one ought to say, this little comedy, for there is nothing really sombre in all these occurrences, will soon be ended.'[33] The completeness of the cure is attested in a footnote to the published lecture.

Charcot gave one more anecdote from his experience. The patient was a girl from Angoulême, aged fourteen, who, after a spurt of rapid adolescent growth, had systematically refused to eat, exemplifying a condition which Charcot said bordered on hysteria without properly belonging to it. 'Nervous anorexia,' had been described in England by Sir William Gull and in France by Lasègue, one of Charcot's predecessors at the Salpêtrière. Such patients are to be distinguished from secret eaters. They have no desire to eat. They eventually become living skeletons and totally weak. Sometimes the will to eat returns too late for their lives to be saved, as they cannot at that stage digest and assimilate.[34] Charcot was first informed of this particular case of anorexia when he received a letter from her father beseeching him to come to Angoulême. Charcot wrote back : 'Bring the child to Paris, place her in a hydropathic establishment, leave her there, or at least when you go away make her believe that you have quitted the capital, inform me of it, and I will do the rest.'[35] One night six weeks later, a medical man from Angoulême arrived in great haste at Charcot's house to say the girl was in a hydropathic clinic in Paris and in extremis. Charcot had not been told because the parents refused to be separated from their daughter. Charcot told him that the sine qua non of the prescription had been misunderstood, but he went to the hydro and found the patient in the final stage of emaciation and already cyanosed.

The little doctor, whose stature did not much exceed sixty inches, took the parents aside and, with the authority of a man ten feet tall, addressed to them what he described as 'a blunt remonstrance.' He said there was but one hope. They must go away, or pretend so, immediately. At last they left, the father 'uttering maledictions.' The results of isolation were 'rapid and marvellous.' The child after a little weeping became '*much less desolate than one would have expected*.' The very same evening, in spite of a repugnance to food, she took a biscuit dipped in wine. At the end of fifteen days she was relatively well, and quite strong and healthy after eight weeks. When Charcot questioned her, she made the following confession :

As long as papa and mama had not gone—in other words, as long as you had not triumphed (for I saw that you wished to shut me up)—I believed that my illness was not serious, and as I had a horror of eating, I did not eat. *But when I saw you were determined to be master, I was afraid*, and in spite of my repugnance I tried to eat, and I was able to, little by little.[36]

Charcot added : 'I thanked the child for her confidence, which, as you will understand, is a lesson in itself.' At the Salpêtrière under Charcot much attention was given to reeducation of the appetite and the alimentary functions. This was done by giving the patients a carefully graduated diet.

Lasègue and, later, Charcot speculated on the psychological causes of anorexia. Charcot, it is said, tended to favor a rather simple (and possibly overly-simple) explanation. He found that one of his anorexic patients wore a rose-coloured ribbon next to her skin and fastened very tightly around the waist. She confided the ribbon was a measure which the waist was not to exceed. 'I prefer dying of hunger to becoming as big as mamma.' Janet comments: 'Coquetries of this kind are very frequent; one of my patients refused to eat for fear that, during digestion, her face should grow red and appear less pleasant in the eyes of a professor whose lectures she attended after her meals.'[37] Janet goes on to suggest that Charcot tended to exaggerate the importance of the consciously held obsessions to anorexic patients, and 'used to seek everywhere for his rose-colored ribbon and the idea of obesity.' Perhaps the little Professor himself was subject to a slight 'phobia' of this sort. Being somewhat of the pyknic type in later life, though he kept his figure reasonably trim, he had a tendency towards *embonpoint* and is likely to have been appreciative of the menace of French cuisine.

At the very end of his life Charcot wrote a booklet on faith healing. This was some eight years after the first edition of Hyppolite Bernheim's book *De la suggestion*. But long prior to 1884, indeed possibly before Bernheim, Charcot had been aware of the subjective element in both the cause and cure of hysterical ailments. Speaking of spontaneous remissions of contracture seen in the Salpêtrière, he said that in former times similar cases were frequently cited as examples of supernatural intervention in therapeutics, and he drew attention to an article by Littre, 'Un fragment de médecine rétrospective,' analyzing several cases of paralysis cured after pilgrimage to the tomb of Saint Louis at St Denis. In respect of three women pilgrims very exact medical details were on record. They each had contractures of the leg with anesthesias. 'You see, gentlemen, things have changed little since the close of the thirteenth century.' Charcot's circle, through their historical researches into hysteria, were interested in a variety of religious *miranda*, such as the excesses of religious enthusiasm and of witch beliefs, ranging from the Jansenist convulsionaries to the possessed nuns of Loudun. Many cases of religious fasting unto death, they remarked, were perhaps related to anorexia. In his book *Science et miracle: Louise Lateau ou la stigmatisée belge*, Bourneville relates a contemporary case of 'stigmatization' to hysterical vasomotor disturbance.[38]

Naturally, also like Bernheim and other medical people, the Salpêterians were aware of the prime religious sensation of nineteenth century France, the rise of Lourdes, rapidly becoming the greatest place of pilgrimage in the Catholic world. The medicinal springs of the Pyrenées were well known to Roman Gaul, whose better-off citizens took their ailing relatives to benefit from thermal baths and to 'take the cure.' The Queen of Navarre (the literary Marguerite) brought her daughter-in-law, Jeanne d'Albret, from Pau to Cauterets, twenty miles from Lourdes, to gain fertility from its waters, and Henry of Navarre in due course was born to greatness. In February 1858, a miller's daughter at Lourdes, the fourteen-year-old Marie-Bernarde Soubirous in the Grotto of Massabielle saw the first of eighteen apparitions of 'The Lady' who gave her name as the 'Immaculate Conception.' Delicate and asthmatic, the future St Bernadette was instructed by the Lady to drink water from the floor of the grotto. With difficulty Bernadette located a tiny trickle, but as she did so a gushing spring broke forth, which is said to yield 27,000 gallons a day. The diocesan and papal authorities, after rather stringent cross-examination and enquiries, eventually authenticated the miracle and in 1864 the pilgrimages were officially approved. Within a decade or so numerous histories of the healings at Lourdes had been written. As early as 1873 Thomas Henry Huxley, visiting France for reasons of health, found one such history on a bookstall in Paris.[39] The challenge of obscurantism (as he thought) aroused him from a profound mental depression and put him in the best of spirits like a warhorse among the trumpets. He proceeded happily to reduce all visions and cures to natural causes, as later on did Bernheim and also the Myers brothers, to say nothing of Zola.[40]

Some time in 1892 Charcot was asked by the *New Review*, an English journal, to give his views on faith healing. He wrote an extremely interesting essay published in January 1893, 'The

Faith-Cure,' which appeared in parallel, as 'La foi qui Guérit,' 'The Faith That Heals,' in the *Archives de neurologie*. After his death it was reprinted in the *Bibliothèque Diabolique*.[41] Except in a very tangential way, Charcot made no reference to Lourdes, but he made use of a remarkable book by Carré de Montgeron, a magnificent production in four volumes,[42] describing in great detail cures effected at St Médard. Janet remarks that those who write of the miracles of Lourdes refer contemptuously to de Montgeron and suggests the reason may be that the book was used as a text by Charcot.[43] But this may not be the full explanation. After all Deacon Pâris, if not exactly a heretic, was a Jansenist and hardly as eligible for canonization as Bernadette. Also enthusiasts for one shrine are not always sedulous in advancing the claims of rival institutions. Lourdes was remarkable only in the degree of its fame and in having its cult first established in modern times. And the latter fact tends to explain the former. The ancients rightly considered Aesculapius immortal, for he never died. Though the god's altars were overturned and his name forgotten, Aesculapian medicine lived on for millennia in the shrines of another religion. Indeed, Christian healing was attached to certain churches before the last pagan clinics were forcibly shut down.[44]

Miracles of healing were not only performed in churches or by the bones of dead saints. Many a humble villager gained celebrity as an effective charmer of warts. Whether he used some herbal salve from folk medicine or the power of his personality, the results were doubtless the same. The kings of France and England had traditionally laid on their hands to cure scrofula, the 'King's-evil.' In the seventeenth century, John Aubrey remarked that this 'does much puzzle our philosophers: for whether our Kings were of the house of York or Lancaster, it did the cure (i.e.) for the most part. 'Tis true indeed at the touching there are prayers read, but perhaps, neither the King attends them nor his chaplains.'[45]

The rebellious son of Lucy Walters and Charles II was never crowned or anointed with the holy oil, yet Aubrey says: 'In Somersetshire, 'tis confidently reported, that some were cured of the King's-evil, by the touch of the Duke of Monmouth; the Lord Chancellor Bacon saith, "That imagination is next kin to miracle-working faith".'[46] Even those with no claim to regality might cure the 'King's-evil.' For Aubrey tells of Samuel Scott, a seventh son of Mr William Scot of Hedington in Wiltshire, who did 'wonderful cures by touching only, viz, as to the King's-evil, wens, etc.' Being the squire's son seems to have helped, for Aubrey remarks that, 'A servant boy of his father's was also a seventh son, but he could do no cures at all.' In the late eighteenth century, a celebrated healer whose cures gained great note was Prince Alexander of Hohenlohe-Waldenberg-Schillingfürst, Archbishop and Grand Provost of Grosswardein in Hungary, and Abbott of St Michael's at Galargia. Hack Tuke observed that 'his name and titles had probably much to do with his influence.'[47]

In 'The Faith that Heals,' Charcot begins by expressing sympathy with the question put to him by the editor of the *New Review*. The physician should not neglect any valid method of cure. 'This is why I have attempted for a long time to discover the underlying mechanism in order to make use of its power.'[48]

But he stressed that healing through faith was a phenomenon belonging to the natural order and could be enquired into by observation and reasoning just like any other scientific problem. The 'miracles' of faith cure had occurred in all times and lands and under the aegis of every religion. On the other hand, its successes were limited; in fact they were confined to those ailments

> whose cure requires no other intervention than the power which the mind possesses over the body. Thus faith will never restore an amputated limb but numerous paralyses yield to it, as do various tumours and ulcers as well as the convulsive seizures of an hysterical nature.[49]

No significant differences can be discerned either in the conditions successfully treated or in the modus operandi in lay faith healing or the religious sphere.

Charcot drew parallels between the most famous Christian shrines and the Aesculapian sanctuaries. The surroundings are frequently the same, fine mountain country, a sacred spring, the dark cave the ancients used to describe as the earth's mouth, and often a wonder-working statue or relics. In an oblique reference to Lourdes, he refers to the servitors of the temple among whom 'are the doctor-priests who are charged with noting and aiding the cures—that is to say the Medical Board which the shrines of today never fail to maintain if they are of sufficient importance.'[50]

Charcot notes the amusing similarity in respect of 'intercessors.' In Greco-Roman times, a patient could employ an intercessor to go to the sanctuary in default of making the journey himself. Charcot found that throughout Poitou there were ladies who could be commissioned by invalids to go on their behalf to the tomb of St Radegonde.

The walls of the Miraculous Grotto at Lourdes are covered with the crutches thrown away by successful pilgrims, and *ex-voto* offerings of every sort. Times change little; the Aesculapian temples were ornamented with votive inscriptions recording the miracles which had been worked. Grateful patients also attached bas-reliefs or small sculptures made of stone, marble, or even silver or gold, representing the parts of the body which had been healed. Only rarely do the reliefs allow of a definite retrospective diagnosis. But Paul Richer described a votive offering that accurately reproduces the position of a foot in a state of hysterical contracture. Charcot turned his diagnostician's eye on the completely similar *ex-voto* marbles set up at modern sanctuaries. He recounts a visit to the venerated Church of St Mary in the Camargue, where he saw among the *ex-voto's* a plaster relief in the shape of the leg of a girl of about twelve years of age, which was deformed as in clubfoot but perfectly reproduced a known form of hysterical contracture. The cure had been rapidly effective and next to the relief a photograph showed the little girl standing squarely on her feet quite free of the contracture.

Charcot then proceeds to the mechanism of the cure by faith. In ordinary circumstances, spontaneous remission does not occur with dramatic force. But often an invalid hears of miraculous cures at a sanctuary, and after much discussion with friends, relatives, and doctors hope arises. At last the resolve to make the journey is formed. This may often involve considerable practical difficulties necessitating thought and preparations. The period of active planning and developing hope is often one of

143

conscious prayer and good works. In short, the pilgrimage is preceded by a period of 'expectation.' Charcot described this period as an 'incubation,' a word suggested by the sleeping-in at the pagan clinics and by his own observation of the phase of *élaboration* between a trauma and the establishment of conversion symptoms. It is in the incubation period that the power of suggestion begins its work, and it is a vital stage in the cure. The invalid eventually arrives at the sanctuary fatigued in body but with heightened belief, and in an eminently suggestible condition. Finally, the fervent prayers, the processions and exalted ceremonies, and perhaps immersion in the sacred water complete their effect and often a cure results. The expectation, the heightened belief, the incubation are essential factors. Local residents are, therefore, not good subjects for miraculous healing, and invalids in the Pyrenées would do best to go to St Médard or St Denis or to Spain.

Charcot then proceeds to an analysis of the illness and cure of Louise Coirin as narrated by Carré de Montgeron. It should be said that de Montgeron was a judge in the Parliament of Paris, and as such was skilled in marshalling evidence. The Demoiselle Coirin was a close relative of an official at the Court of Louis XV, and de Montgeron was well placed to obtain a detailed account of her symptoms. An unmarried lady aged thirty-one living at Nanterre (a village just across the Seine from Neuilly), she was thrown from her horse in 1716. Forty days later she passed into a state of weakness with hemorrhage. Two months later her left breast had become swollen, hard, and violet in color. Fomentations and local bleeding had no effect and cancer was diagnosed. But the patient did not die. Instead, in 1718 she became paralyzed in the whole of her left side with contracture of the arm and leg which were cold to the touch.

An amputation of the now profoundly ulcerated breast was refused in 1720 and the Demoiselle remained in the same dolorous condition until 1731, when resort was had to saintly intervention. On August 9, 1731, a local lady was asked to say a *novena* on Demoiselle Coirin's behalf at the tomb of M de Pâris at St Médard. The patient then was taken in person to the sanctuary, but her condition permitted of only a few hours' stay. However, on the evening of August 11 she applied to her affected side and breast a shift that had lain in contact with the tomb of Deacon François. On August 12 the same was done with some of the precious earth from St Médard churchyard. The ulcer immediately started to dry up. On August 13 the paralyzed arm became warm and mobile, and the contracture of the left leg relaxed. The Demoiselle now could raise herself in bed, put her toes to the ground, and dress herself. The miracle proceeded. Three days had been enough to relieve the paralyses, the contractures, and circulatory inhibition. But it was only on September 24 that the wounds on her breast were fully closed and cicatrized.

Charcot observes that he had for ten years past drawn attention to hysterical hemorrhages, paralyses, and contractures. But was the 'cancer' of the breast also hysterical? In answer he notes the frequency of neurotic persistent ulcerations, as in the stigmatic Louise Lateau.[51] Louise Coirin's breast, said Charcot, was the site of a hysterical edema, a condition first mentioned by Sydenham and described in Gilles de la Tourette's treatise. A paper by the English physician Fowler on 'Neurotic Tumours of the Breast' (1890) should also be noted. Fowler advised the introduction of a psychic element into the treatment of these conditions which were distinguishable from malignant ones requiring surgery. In letters to Charcot, Fowler had reported spontaneous cures exactly similar to those accomplished through religious faith.

Unlike Bertrin, who wrote a best-selling treatise on the apparitions and cures at Lourdes, Charcot was not worried as to whether the Virgin Mary ought to leave a scar when she heals miraculously.[52] Even faith healing, he said, follows the laws of nature. Though a contracture might be suddenly relieved, the limb would show diminished sensibility and exaggerated tendon reflexes for some days after. It is a physiologic law that these phenomena cannot disappear immediately. As he had often demonstrated at the Salpêtrière, where they had cures as dramatic as at any sanctuary, subsequent to the initial drama, physiological repair and renewal took their natural course. Louise Coirin's edema had cleared up rapidly in accordance with the well-established fact that circulatory troubles often disappear suddenly. Repair of the tissues could then proceed by natural healing processes, but this took its full time—six weeks. It was seven weeks before atrophy of the leg had diminished sufficiently to allow her to mount her carriage.

Charcot concluded by stressing that maladies successfully cured by faith need special subjects—subjects especially prone to *autosuggestion*. He ends on a cautious note, paraphrasing his favorite author:

> Is it to say that already at present we know everything in the domain of the supernatural contribution to faith-healing; and shall we see its frontiers always retreating under the influence of the growth of secular knowledge? Certainly not! It is necessary while always seeking to know how to wait. I am always the first to acknowledge that today
> > There are more things in heaven and earth
> > Than are dreamt of in thy philosophy.[53]

CHAPTER VI

Metals and Magnets

CHARCOT, LIKE many of his illustrious compeers in the Faculty of Medicine such as Brouardel and some of his associates such as Bourneville, was a freethinker. But this group, like their contemporary, Bernheim, did not approach the 'miracles' wrought by the 'occult' or the 'supernatural' in a spirit of crude or crass materialism. They differed from the more mechanistic type of physician who, failing to find an organic lesion when examining a hysteric or a hypochondriac, classified the patient as a *malade imaginaire* and would then tell him to be less fanciful and not think so much about his health. Such a 'common-sense down-to-earth' attitude is otiose, because it turns its back on causal medicine and fails to ask, 'Why?' Why does such a patient believe himself ill? As the Charcot school put it, a disease induced by the workings of the imagination is not an imaginary disease, but is as 'real' as any other ailment. They were aware of Lasègue's aphorism 'not everyone who pleases can be hypochondriac.' Consequently the attitude of the Salpêtrière school, like that of Nancy, to religious miracles was one of enlightened acceptance of the reality of the cures. The coarser sceptics denied not so much the reality of the cures, as the reality of the disease. But as a large part of Charcot's scientific work had been directed at establishing the reality of neuroses, this was a line of argument which the Salpêtrians could hardly have taken even if they had so wished. Indeed, in respect of the genuineness of such cures as were affected by apparently transcendental means, the Salpêtrians were somewhat on the side of the religious, the faith healers, and the mesmerists.

Charcot's distinguished pupils Féré (Assistant Physician at the

Salpêtrière) and Alfred Binet (later Director of the psychological laboratory at the Sorbonne and in due time one of the most eminent of psychologists) said in their valuable book *Animal Magnetism* that 'those who undertake miraculous cures' act very differently from the physician who tells his patient that it is all in the imagination and that he shouldn't stuff his head with things he doesn't understand. The miraculous healers

> do not deny the existence of the disease, but they assert that it may be cured by supernatural power. They act by means of suggestion, and by gradually inculcating the idea that the disease is curable, until the subject accepts it. The cure is sometimes effected by the suggestion, and when it is said to be by 'saving faith,' the expression used is rigorously scientific. These miracles should no longer be denied but we should understand their genesis and learn to imitate them.[1]

The last sentence is practically a quotation from Charcot's *La foi qui guérit*, which had not been written when Binet and Féré published their book, and we can conclude that it was a standing dictum at the Salpêtrière. In their Preface to *Animal Magnetism*, the authors say :

> We think it well to state that this work was written in the environment of the Salpêtrière. By this we not only mean that our descriptions apply to facts observed in that hospital, but also that our personal observations were made in accordance with the method inaugurated by M. Charcot, the chief of the school of the Salpêtrière, . . .[2]

Their views can therefore be taken as thoroughly representative of Salpêtrian beliefs in the early 1880's and it is clear that, just as is evidenced by Charcot's own lectures, the power of suggestion was very considerably appreciated in the hospital. It is useful to stress this, because many modern histories of psychiatrics and related topics tend to convey an impression that 'suggestion' was a mystery withheld from Charcot and a discovery first unveiled by Bernheim in 1884.

We should try to imitate miracles, said Charcot—in effect.

But, as we have seen, he pointed out that the resources of the physician are more scanty than those of the thaumaturge, when it comes to deploying suggestion on a grand scale. But occasionally the physician can assist the patient's own automatism to arrive at a supernatural cure even in a strictly clinical environment. Here it is pleasing to note the later history of Justine Etch. mentioned earlier as a chronic invalid consequent on a sexual trauma.

> When a believer associates the Deity with his idea of cure, he is accustomed to expect it to be sudden and complete, as the result of a definite religious manifestation; and this, in fact, often occurs. We had a well known instance at the Salpêtrière, when a woman of the name of Etchverry was, after her devotions in the month of May, suddenly cured of an hemiplegia and contracture by which she had been affected for seven years. Only a slight weakness of the side remained, which disappeared in a few days, and which could be explained by the prolonged inaction of the muscles. This may be termed an experimental miracle, since the physicians had prepared for it beforehand, having for a long time previously suggested to the subject that she would be cured when a certain religious ceremony took place. . . .[3]

We need not suppose that Charcot and his associates, being of the profession of Rabelais and hence tending toward a minimal degree of devoutness, specially indoctrinated Justine in the religion of saving grace. It is likely that suggestion was applied more indirectly by way of repeated assertions that her condition was progressing and that a cure was certain, and that she would be well by her saint's day (which is probably the religious occasion referred to). Doubtless, this oblique suggestion was reinforced with anecdotes concerning miraculous cures.

'Medicine for the imagination' (as Binet and Féré felicitously put it) explicitly occupied an important place in the battery of therapeutic methods deployed at the Salpêtrière. As Binet and Féré also point out, suggestion accounted in large degree for the beneficial effects of most of the other treatments—isolation, hydrotherapy, and electrotherapy—a fact of which their master was equally aware, if not more so. The range of treatments administered on Charcot's service was extensive. On occasion this has been made a ground of criticism, presumably as indicating a tolerance of empirical rather than causal medicine. But Charcot might have retorted that, he had to do his best for his patients, and that he was obliged to try anything that was not actually harmful, and that if a causal approach was possible, would his critic be good enough to indicate it. As Charcot had done as much as any man of his time to define hysteria and analyze its etiology, this imaginary dialogue (which may perhaps on occasion have taken place in reality) would be brought to a somewhat conclusive termination. Nonetheless, Charcot's eclecticism in the matter of treatments has not failed to earn him reproach from some medical historians. This criticism relates especially to metallotherapy and the use of magnets. Somewhat paradoxically, in respect of hypnosis Charcot is criticized from a contrary direction; namely, for having taken too narrow a 'research view,' and he is censured for reluctance to employ hypnosis on a large scale in therapeutics.

Charcot's fate in connection with metals and magnetism, animal or mineral, illustrates rather neatly the dilemma of the scientist. Should he be open-minded and take a broad view of possibilities, he is called uncritical. Yet, if he restricts himself to 'fundamental research,' he is liable to be accused of indifference to human need. But this dilemma is, of course, only one facet of the problem as to whether and precisely how in the person of Charcot, Homer did nod, and this question is a complex one. Janet was the last writer to deal with it at all illuminatingly, and subsequent historians have dealt with it in a rather facile manner, tending to repeat over-briefly the polemics of the 'School of Nancy.' Professor Guillain of the Salpêtrière is an honorable exception, but he was handicapped by lack of space for full discussion in his otherwise excellent book.[4] Of Axel Munthe we shall speak later. The question of Charcot's errors, real or alleged, is—like many others in psychology—not entirely a simple one. Nor can it be solved expeditiously or reliably with the wisdom of hindsight. It must be fitted into the entire complex constituted by nineteenth-century ideas of magnetism, electrobiology, physics, and psychophysiology. Consequently, the task of just appraisal is not to be adequately met by either of the simple alternatives of sending for a bucket of whitewash or, contrariwise, shouting 'Off with his head!'

Metallotherapy entered the Salpêtrière in 1876, about the same time as Charcot's attention was being drawn to hypnotism. Although Mesmer came from Austria and the word *hypnotism* was adapted from Greek *hypnos* (sleep) by James Braid, a Scotsman, France above all others was the 'metropolis' of animal magnetism. The lodestone may have been used as an amulet against disease in ancient Egypt, and metal plates were used in cure by Perkins in the United States at the end of the eighteenth century as recounted by Oliver Wendell Holmes,[5] but in the nineteenth century France was the true home of metallotherapy, iron plates being attached to the wrists or chests of his patients by the Abbé Lenoble, and magnets being used in treatment by physicians as celebrated as Laennec and Trousseau. Some of the mesmerists (i.e., the 'animal magnetizers') adopted these ideas relating to the efficacy of metals, ferromagnetic and otherwise. In his treatise of 1840, *De l'emploi du magnétisme animal et des eaux minérales dans le traitement des maladies nerveuses*, Charles Despine wrote, apropos of his famous hysterical patient Estelle:

> I was struck by the remarkable fondness which these patients had for pure gold; I also noted the obviously different influences exercised upon them by zinc, brass and magnetized iron. . . . As soon as the brass touched her, it undid the good effects of the gold.[6]

The subject was then taken up in a big way by Victor Burq, who in 1851 devoted his doctoral thesis to it and wrote many papers subsequently, as well as a treatise *Des origines de la metallothérapie* in 1883.[7] Burq's efforts were always applied to the restoration of sensibility in the anesthetic limbs of hysterical patients. He regarded the anesthesia as the foundation of the hysterical syndrome and the basic measure of the intensity of the disease. His method was to put a bracelet consisting of linked plaques of the same metal onto the anesthetic forearm. (This was the treatment received by Dum. from his own physician when he left the Salpêtrière.) If the metal had been favorably chosen, the subject would experience the return of sensation, progressing from tingling and sense of heat and weight in the limb to 'pins and needles' all over his skin. This heralded the return of sensibility to all parts of the body, and often complete relief of paralyses. Sometimes the patient's tendency to convulsive attacks also disappeared.

In 1876 Burq submitted his experimental findings to the Society of Biology, which appointed a commission to examine his claims. As President of the Commission, Charcot had the experiments repeated at the Salpêtrière. His research workers and interns took to them with enthusiasm. They soon confirmed that relief of anesthetic and other symptoms could be effected in some patients by Burq's method. In addition, they established more definitely than Burq had indicated that recoveries from anesthesia tended to be temporary only, there being a strong tendency for the patient to revert to local insensibility. Bourneville, Paul Richer, and Dumontpallier were among the enthusiasts for metallotherapy. With each individual patient the research went through the stage of *metalloscopy*, which consisted in trials of various metals until, if possible, one should be found which was efficacious with that patient. Despine's Estelle, like Danaë, responded best to gold, but some patients did better with copper or iron. It was discovered further that various other agents could be equally effective, for example, tuning forks, magnets, blister poultices, electric currents, and static electricity. These findings were summarized in articles by Romain Vigouroux, in which he said that Charcot had applied the term *aesthesiogenic* to all these agents: 'The name of *aesthesiogenism* is the general term proposed by Charcot to denote all the natural agents or processes which, like metals, have a special action upon sensation and certain other functions.'[8]

Among these discoveries was the phenomenon of *transfer* first found by Gellé during the aesthesiogenic treatment of a patient with hysterical deafness. At the moment when hearing had become normal on the side of the hemianesthesia, the patient became deaf in the other ear! This was soon verified to be a common result with limb anesthesias, paralyses and hysterical disorders of vision. Charcot's favorite aesthesiogen was the magnet. In his lectures he remarked sometimes of a patient that application of a magnet had produced a *transfer* and that this was hopeful, because at the Salpêtrière they had found that repeated transfers from one side to the other often led to a reduced intensity of symptoms, and thus to a complete or partial cure. Professor Guillain accedes to the popular modern view of metallotherapy and magnetotherapy when he says, in effect, that the observations on aesthesiogenism were faulty. 'For a description of these mechanisms he [i.e., Charcot] relied on investigations pursued by collaborators whose competence in neurology and psychiatry was open to question.'[9] But this is not quite the whole story. There is no doubt that the effects on the patients, transfers or induced cures, were genuinely observed. Where Charcot's assistants, and perhaps he himself, went astray was in believing that these effects derived from physical forces exerted by the magnet or by the metal plates.

This may seem a little naïve to us, but we must judge it in relation to the biophysics of the time. Burq's own hypothesis was not unreasonable. He supposed the influence to consist in the slight electric currents that in fact are produced by contact of a metal with the skin. In this he was followed by Paul Régnard (coauthor with Bourneville of *The Iconography of the Salpêtrière*), and Pitres, one of Charcot's junior collaborators, who became professor at Bordeaux. However, there were serious objections to theories of this sort. It seems in general that it is not only necessary for the aesthesiogen to be applied, but that the patient has to be aware that it is being employed. Vigouroux himself set up an experiment using an electromagnet operated by an assistant in another room who would switch it on and off unbeknown to the patient. According to Janet whenever he, Janet, carried out the experiment, no transfer or aesthesiogenic effect occurred, though it did with Vigouroux. Janet's opinion, was that the experiment was set up in an insufficiently rigorous way; that is, the subject was able consciously or subconsciously to infer from various clues when the magnet was switched on.[10] If extrasensory perception is left out of account as being at most only very exceptionally in operation, it follows that the favorable reactions of subjects to aesthesiogens were not to be correctly explained through the virtues of the aesthesiogens, but in purely psychological terms.

The psychological mechanism is itself not to be simply understood. It is not merely a suggestive reaction to the magnet, or bottle of iron filings, or the gold plate itself. It was frequently noted that with the same subject and the same aesthesiogen, a positive result is achieved when the treatment is applied by one physician but not when employed by another. Janet says that the magnet produced wonderful cures and alleviations in the period around 1880, but that ten years later when he was at the Salpêtrière he could get no effects with it.[11] In 1886 Bernheim produced his famous book *La Suggestion* (a second and expanded version of his book of 1884) in which, among other things, he proposed that all the aesthesiogenic effects were the result of suggestions.[12] This led, for the most part, to a complete abandonment of aesthesiogenics, except insofar as it may still have been used for treatment at the Salpêtrière. Bernheim, of course, accepted the reality of the effects. But once the purely psychological nature of the effects had been asserted, the aesthesiogenists lost heart and the subject disappeared as a field for research and theory.

The reality of transfer in particular was attested by Freud in the preface he wrote to his own translation into German of Bernheim's book. He also counters the hypotheses advanced by Hüchel in 1888 concerning the origin of transfer. Hüchel supposed that transfer was originally suggested, consciously or unconsciously, to some particular hysterical patient and that as a result of this early example, physicians ever since have continued to produce this symptom by suggestion. If this were true of transfer, why should it not be true of all the other hysterical symptoms? Freud remarks:

But the principal points of the symptomatology of hysteria are safe from the suspicion of having originated from suggestion by a physician. Reports coming from past times and from distant lands, which have been collected by Charcot and his pupils, leave no room for doubt that the peculiarities of hysterical attacks, of hysterogenic zones, of anaesthesias, paralyses and contractures, have been manifested at every time and place just as they were at the Salpêtrière when Charcot carried out his memorable investigation of that major neurosis.[13]

Apart from this reductio ad absurdum, Freud said that transfer occurs spontaneously in cases of hysteria uninfluenced by suggestion. Janet describes such a case:

> I was seeking one day to cure a small localized symptom, to restore the motion of the right wrist with a patient whose fist was contractured. . . . This work [i.e., re-education after the method of Charcot] is long and troublesome. . . . When it had proceeded for some time, the result seemed marvellous; the right hand had opened and moved freely in every way; the patient left the laboratory very happy and proud. She re-entered it a few moments later in despair. 'It was not worth while making such efforts,' she said, presenting her left fist, which was contractured exactly in the same way as her right fist had been a few minutes before. I have cited this episode because it struck me by the circumstances in which it occurred; namely in a quite naïve patient, having no notion of the phenomenon, and without the operator or herself having had the least idea of it beforehand.[14]

Some words of Freud's in the article already quoted would seem to be applicable to this kind of experience, even though he did in fact use them in relation to other neurotic reactions (the reflex hyperexcitability discovered by Charcot in hypnotized hystericals at the Salpêtrière):

> . . . it is a question in these cases not so much of suggestions as of stimulation to *autosuggestions*. And these as anyone can see, contain an objective factor, independent of the physician's will, and they reveal a connection between various conditions, of innervation or excitation in the nervous system. It is autosuggestions such as these that lead to the production of spontaneous hysterical paralyses and it is an inclination to such autosuggestions rather than suggestibility which, from the point of view of the physician, characterizes hysteria; nor do the two seem by any means to run parallel.[15]

Freud went on to say that in fact Bernheim himself worked with indirect suggestions—that is, with stimulations to auto-suggestions: 'suggestion pushes open the doors which are in fact slowly opening of themselves by auto-suggestion.'[16]

Janet, when recounting his experience of spontaneous transfer of contracture of the hand, goes on to assimilate this phenomenon to the general tendency of conversion hysterics to substitute one symptom for another—'the disposition to *equivalences*,' as he calls it:

Hysteria, in fact, is a very singular malady, the cure of which one never dares to assert. It is often easy, through some psychological process or other, to cause such or such a determinate symptom to disappear. Besides, these symptoms often disappear of themselves in consequence of an emotion, of some upset, or even without [apparent] reason. But when a symptom has disappeared, especially when it has disappeared too quickly, we should not at once cry out victory. First of all the same symptom is very likely soon to reappear. Then the following strange thing very frequently occurs: another apparently quite different symptom takes the place of the first.[17]

Janet exemplifies this substitution by the case history of a girl of twelve, anorexic with uncontrollable nausea and vomiting. He cured the vomiting by aesthesiogenic treatment (probably electricity) and got her to eat regularly. 'This seems all right but from that moment this girl, till then perfectly intelligent, enters into a state of mental confusion and delirium, and it becomes impossible to stop this delirium without the vomitings beginning again.[18] There are numerous instances of symptom substitution. For example, mental disturbances can substitute for contractures and vice versa; contractures can alternate with mutism. In his lectures Charcot drew attention to the fact that the onset of a paralysis is often correlated with a complete cessation of previous hysterical attacks and thus appears to substitute for the attacks. Transfer is therefore to be understood as a reflection of the fact that the symptoms of conversion hysteria are valuable to the affected subject who has an unconscious disposition to hang on to them. Transfer is a particularly simple kind of substitution, because it replaces the original symptom by an extremely similar one, one that is both psychologically and physically almost identical.

Transfer, symptom substitution, and also more or less complete cures effected apparently by the use of magnets or plates were reported not only by the Salpêtrians and their associates such as Dumontpallier at the Hôtel-Dieu hospital in Paris, but by other workers such as Ladame in Geneva, and they must be counted as genuine phenomena. The reality of transfer is also attested in a different context where aesthesiogens were not used. The 'magnetizers' such as Cabanis (i.e., the mesmerists operating only with 'animal magnetism') had noted that sometimes the sensibility on the two sides of the body behaved in their patients 'like a fluid, its level lowering on one side when it rises on the other.' Even after most other workers had forsaken metallotherapy, Sollier brought out a book in 1897 giving a psychological study of twenty hysterical patients and the results of aesthiogenic treatment.[19] Sollier found that under prolonged aesthiogenic treatment, some of his subjects would show a return to complete health. However, these cures were rarely permanent and relapses were the rule. But if the course of aesthesiogenic treatment were repeated, the subsequent relapse was often less acute. Sollier claimed that, after the application of a few cycles of treatment and subsequent relapse, half the patients stayed cured for periods of one or of several years, half remained well for some months, and the remainder showed marked amelioration of symptoms. Jules and Pierre Janet had a rather similar experience with aesthesiogens a few years earlier.[20]

Pierre Janet, however, while at Le Havre and then later at the Salpêtrière, had obtained many of these transformations by other means. These patients were usually acute hysterics with a variety of symptoms. Janet reports :

Wishing to work simultaneously towards the curing of these patients and towards elucidating the pathogenesis of their symptoms, I tried by all possible means to modify these symptoms, to dispel them by hypnotism, by suggestion, and by various educational methods. I endeavoured to make the paralysed limbs resume the power of proper movement; to induce the patients to feel and to appreciate the impressions made upon their dulled senses.

In some of my patients, and especially in three of them, this practice led to the onset of conditions which seemed to me very strange, for they were in complete contrast with the habitual morbid condition. Sometimes these states appeared gradually, after the subjects had been making efforts to move and to feel, and they were preceded by contortions, and by itching or other forms of dysaesthesia. In most cases they appeared in the course of a hypnotic sitting, and after a period of profound sleep. In particular they were characterized by the complete disappearance of *all* the pathological phenomena.[21]

These patients were to all intents and purposes well, not only physically but in mind. There were no disorders of will, and suggestibility had apparently disappeared. Janet christened this state one of *complete somnambulism*: 'This final condition of somnambulism is a state in which the subject, whose personality has hitherto been so greatly restricted, and who in the waking state was so ill, has now become identical with one who is perfectly well and completely normal.'[22] It may seem strange that Janet regarded this healthy state as one of complete somnambulism, but he explains the matter as follows:

In my first studies of this question I was at great pains to show that this state was not in itself in any way extra-ordinary; that it was simply the normal condition in which these women ought to have been all the time. . . . I was sorry to find, . . . that the condition of complete restoration was one which could not last long in these patients. If they were left to themselves, they relapsed sooner or later. . . . Another and very important phenomenon now attracted my attention in connexion with these cases. I found that the patients, when they had relapsed into their habitual morbid state, had as a rule completely forgotten the period of artificially induced health. These oblivions made gaps in the continuity of memory thus giving birth to various modifications of the personality. That is why, in order to denote the periods of temporary restoration, I use the term 'complete somnambulism,' which had already been employed by Azam to denote kindred phenomena.[23]

Janet noted also that these transformations closely resembled the 'magnetic crises' described by Charles Despine in Estelle's case. Estelle, though completely paralyzed in her 'waking state,' was fit enough to swim and even give swimming lessons in the 'somnambulistic state.'[24]

The transformation from a multisymptomatic hysterical state to that of 'complete somnambulism' is, of course, a phenomenon different from symptom substitution or transfer. First brought to the attention of the medical world in the person of 'Félida X,' Dr Azam's patient, complete somnambulism was but one among a great variety of abnormal mental states either found in patients or developed in them under hypnotic or other treatment. At the Salpêtrière, they were very familiar with patients brought in subsequent to somnambulistic fugues. The fugue represents the typical case of 'loss of memory'—the man who ups and leaves his home and place of work to wander far in an unusual state of consciousness. Sometimes the peculiarity of the mental state is outwardly hardly perceptible even to the trained observer, but often these patients exhibit abstractness or vagueness in such extreme degree that Charcot used to say it was a marvel that such people were not stopped before they boarded the railway train.[25] One of Charcot's own notable achievements was to recognize the somnambulistic character of the phase of the *attitudes passionnelles* in hysterical attacks. This state is not really distinct in nature from the somnambulistic fugue. The patient is in no sense asleep; he lives in a dream of his own and, though physically and mentally active, is relatively indifferent to external reality. The state of the *attitudes passionnelles* in some degree is also akin to somnambulism as encountered in everyday life (the layman's meaning of the term)—sleepwalking episodes in adults and more frequently in children, in which awareness of the environment is partial and selective to an extent varying from person to person.

Over the years a variety of somnambulistic states was observed at the Salpêtrière and elsewhere, notably by the brothers Jules and Pierre Janet. Jules started his medical career as an intern at La Pitié. Pierre, born in Paris in 1859, took after his uncle Paul Janet, whom he describes not merely as a philosopher interested in mind but as a 'spiritual metaphysician' and 'a great spirit who was interested also in politics and the sciences, and who with great liberalism, sought to reunite these studies. He understood the importance of medical and anatomical studies to the moral intelligence of man.'[26] Pierre Janet studied at the École Normale and then, through the good offices of Uncle Paul, was introduced to the physiological laboratory at the Sorbonne. At the instance of his uncle, Pierre enrolled at the Medical School and undertook to combine medical and philosophical studies. About 1882, Pierre went to Le Havre to teach philosophy at the Lycée. Despite his official duties, he was enabled by the courtesy of Dr Powilewicz to pursue observations in medical psychology at the local hospital. His aim at that time was to write a dissertation on the mechanism of perception as deduced from a study of hallucinations, and he enquired of a local medical practitioner, Dr Gibert, as to availability of hallucinated subjects. Gibert knew of none, but put Janet in contact with a former patient who, in his opinion, was psychologically very remarkable. This was Léonie, who, says Pierre Janet,

had been hypnotized in her youth by Dr Perrier of Caen, who had been introduced by Dupotet, and who had been observed to perform some curious things with clairvoyance, mental suggestion, and hypnotism from a distance etc. What a godsend for a young psychologist, 22 years of age, curious as to all psychological phenomena and drawn by the mysterious side of these occult faculties! At my request Gibert had the celebrated Léonie brought to Le Havre and my studies on her at various periods over a stretch of years oriented my early works towards the marvels of hypnotic somnambulism.[27]

Pierre Janet's first experiments, which concerned 'telepathic hypnotization' (*sommeil à distance*) seemed to him if not entirely conclusive, nevertheless 'quite strange and worthy of attention and discussion.' He submitted a little paper on the results to the Society of Physiological Psychology which had been founded in 1885, having Charcot as its president, Charles Richet as its secretary, and Paul Janet and Professor Théodule Ribot as vice-presidents. Pierre was thus well placed to attract the attention of Charcot. The introduction was reinforced by Pierre Janet's very significant book on somnambulisms, *L'automatisme psychologique,* which appeared in 1889—the same year that the Charcot-Richet society organized the first congress of psychology. At the end of that year Charcot summoned Janet to Paris to supervise the psychological laboratory at the Salpêtrière, the latest addition to the facilities which Charcot had taken such pride in adding to his *service.* Janet's relations with *le patron* were cordial and uncontroversial, as evidenced by his next book, *The Mental State of Hystericals,* published in 1892. During the same period, Charcot lectured on somnambulism and multiple personality in hysterics, particularly in a Salpêtrière patient named Marie Hablon, and Georges Guinon produced a long review of the same subject.[28]

In his own book, Pierre Janet passes over in silence the controversial features of Salpêtrian *major hypnosis and reflex hyperexcitability,* but no other criticism of Salpêtrian attitudes is made overtly or implied by omission. Indeed, the book quotes numerous remarks and dicta of Charcot's. It is full of material drawn from observations made by Janet himself at the Salpêtrière and by other Salpêtrians. Janet's book also reveals that, to a surprising degree, the philosopher-psychologist and the clinical neuropathologist approached the facts of observation in a similiar way and tended to conclusions that were broadly coincident. Charcot wrote a preface:

> I am happy to recommend to the medical public the book of one of my pupils, M. Pierre Janet, on the mental state of hystericals. These studies, begun a long time ago, have been completed in my *service* and set forth in a few lectures which M. Janet delivered this spring at the Salpêtrière. They confirm a thought often expressed in our lectures, namely, that hysteria is largely a mental malady. This is one of the features of this malady we should never neglect if we wish to understand and treat it.
>
> M. Pierre Janet wished to unite as completely as possible medical studies with philosophical studies; it was necessary to bring together these two kinds of knowledge and these two edu-

cations in an effort to analyse clinically the mental state of a patient.[29]

It is somewhat misleading, therefore, to say with Zilboorg that although Janet is frequently classed among the adherents to the 'School of the Salpêtrière,' 'in actuality he was far removed from it and did not belong to the Charcot group.' It is true that not having trained within the group, Janet came to it with his own knowledge and fund of ideas. But it would be unfair to Charcot not to recognize how many explicatory phrases that we nowadays associate primarily with Janet were used earlier by Charcot in his own expositions. Janet's book and Charcot's preface point to a harmonious community of mind between the elder and the younger savant, and Zilboorg is more correct when he says that 'Janet's attitude towards his psychological findings was almost the same as Charcot's towards his clinical observations.'[30]

To revert to the metallotherapic cures and transfers: it is difficult to resist Janet's conclusion that these are instances of transformation of mental states apt to arise spontaneously in the therapeutic situation, and that they are unrelated to the physical properties peculiar to the particular aesthesiogen. After 1885, followers of Bernheim explained the cures and transfers rather facilely as results of 'suggestion.' *Suggestion* is very convenient as a broad description connoting the totality of psychological influences bearing on the patient but, as often pointed out in the subsequent controversies, 'suggestion' is an unanalyzed term. Of course, the conditions at the Salpêtrière were quite conducive to the transmission of direct suggestions even when unintended. Though very far from being a 'snake-pit,' like the public asylums in some of the obscurer regions of even the Western world, the Salpêtrière lacked the spacious colonnades of 'Blair General' or the great modern hospitals of the mid-twentieth century. It was a crowded, intimate place. Despite all efforts at expansion and amenity, physicians, interns, research workers, nursing staff, and patients milled around together at close range. 'It is perhaps not beautiful here,' said Charcot as he showed the visitor around his domain, 'but you can find room for everything you want to do.'[31] And they certainly found room for all manner of researches, but the conditions were not quite as austere as experimental psychology—a discipline then unborn —would prefer. Surprises and 'happenings' were not infrequent:

A man Sm. is completely paraplegic for several months. He is brought on a stretcher into M. Charcot's office. There a violent attack of hysteria develops; he drags himself on the floor, then gradually, controlled by a dream, he gets up, opens the door, and runs as fast as he can through the hospital . . . he climbs up a spout, with wonderful skill, and takes refuge on the roof.[32]

But more seriously for the evaluation of observations was the fact that many of the experimenters, at least in the early days, had little idea that they were dealing with psychological phenomena and, in the words of Janet,

[failed] to understand that their first business should have been to study the mental condition of the subject, and that all kinds of moral precautions were essential . . . thought only of the physical aspects of their experiments. . . . They correctly weighed the metallic plates in chemical balances, and they registered the most trifling muscular tremors with the aid of Marey's tambour; but they saw nothing wrong in carrying on the experiments in public amid the chatter of casual spectators, and they would themselves discuss the meaning of the experiments in their patients' presence.[33]

Naturally, the nurses and the other patients would also convey the general drift of what was being done. A hospital, especially one with so many chronic patients—'old hands'—as the Salpêtrière, where in addition the atmosphere (if not precisely Latin) was a good deal less restrictive than in most asylums and a considerable degree of liberty and mobility was rightly accorded to the patients (by the nature of their ailments, not all bedridden), is as conducive to gossip as any institution in the world. Yet, whether suggestion was direct or indirect, it does not alter the objective factual nature of the symptom transfers and transformations obtained. Indeed, we can easily see that in a sense, part of the efficacy of the theoretically faulty but practically operative metallotherapeutic methods resulted from their 'gimmicky' nature. In an age that has come to recognize the persuasive power of the gimmick this is perhaps more obvious than formerly. In Charcot's day the magnet, though not a rarity, was less mundane than it is now, when any child knows that there is a magneto in every internal combustion engine. An electromagnet was even more prestigious. A patient in whom religious faith was feeble might yet find the new-fangled devices of science numinous and possessed of *mana*.

The rudiments of saving faith could thus be present in the most infidel breast. But the rudiments are not enough without *élaboration*. As with faith cures, there must be a period of preparation in which hope, expectation, and heightened belief can be matured. Just as the pilgrims to the shrines are conditioned by the talk of the priests and their fellow supplicants, so the shop talk of the physicians and the chatter of the patients at the Salpêtrière may have set the stage for transfers and transformations. The atmosphere of the Salpêtrière has been criticized for being somewhat dramatic and excitable. This accusation certainly has some factual basis. Of the savants who came and went in Professor Charcot's *service*, Pierre Marie and Charles Bouchard were on the prim side, but extrovert enthusiasts of all ages participated in the work. Charcot's comrades-in-arms of long standing included men of the cast of Broca and Bourneville who can only be described as men of commitment—intellectual firebrands, eager and dashing. Bramwell, after visiting Liébeault's clinic in 1889, contrasted in his book *Hypnotism* the rustic idyll of proceedings at Nancy with 'the picture drawn by Binet and Féré [in *Animal Magnetism*] of the morbid excitement shown at the Salpêtrière.' This, admittedly, was said specifically with reference to work in hypnotism. But (if we discount or suspend judgment on the possibly gratuitous intensive, morbid) we can take it as evidence of a notable degree of enthusiasm among Charcot's coworkers—a fervor quite likely to be slightly repellent to an Englishman whose race, it must be confessed, tends to regard enthusiasm as superheated or perfervid if it is too overtly expressed.

'Suggestion,' direct or more subtle, is thus a somewhat inadequate word to apply to what has to be regarded as response to the total psychological atmosphere in which patients found themselves. The situation might differ in many respects from the somewhat sentimental charm of Lourdes but its impact, though effective less frequently than at the mountain shrine, nonetheless might on occasion act with equal power. As Charcot said in his essay on cures by faith : *'Les siècles ont passé, mais la source sacrée coule toujours.'* 'The centuries have gone by, but the sacred spring still flows.' To such a situation we can apply a phrase used by Charcot in his lecture on 'Spiritualism and Hysteria,' 'Whatever forcibly strikes the mind, whatever strongly impresses the imagination, is singularly favourable in subjects predisposed. . . .'[34] The sacred spring could be replaced by a bottle of tap water if only the imagination were susceptible and the stage had been appropriately set. Indeed Dr Luys at the Charité hospital obtained transfers and cures by showing the patients bottles of medicine, a treatment that came into ridicule after Bernheim made his criticisms. This is not to say that Bernheim's criticisms were not timely for, as Janet observes, 'His great merit was that he made doctors realise the risk of suggestion, and the need for a psychological analysis if they wished to interpret neuropathic symptoms.'[35] When, as we have done here, we minimize the significance of direct suggestion, we have no wish to defend the Salpêtrians from the charge of having made an intellectual error that, in the early days, did cause them to misinterpret the effects of aesthesiogens so that they referred these effects to actual physical forces—magnetic, electric, or what you will——radiating from the aesthesiogenic substances. Their mode of work, in the teeming warren of the Salpêtrian wards and clinics, allowed every form of suggestion to be inadvertently communicated to the subjects. Janet is right when he sums up the matter thus, with reference to the return of color vision in hysterical achromatopsia :

Vigouroux said in former days that *transfer* could not be a phenomenon of suggestion, because the subject could not possibly have in his head Landolt's law concerning the order in which colours disappear when the visual field is reduced . . . these things seemed to them to be too complex to be the outcome of suggestion. Now, we know today (1925) that they are wrong. A subject who lives in a hospital where people are always talking about such matters is likely to know better than most medical students the order of the colours prescribed by Landolt's law. . . . A suggestion may be extremely complex, so that one single sign, awakening a tendency rich in associations, may bring about multiform reactions.[36]

But the fact remains that 'suggestion' is not a simple concept. If it were less subtle and complex, the practice of healing neurotics would be much simplified. The physician would only need to repeat, 'You are getting better, your cure is certain.' If simple suggestion were all, the cure rate at the Salpêtrière would have been 100 per cent among their hysterics. But of 'suggestion' Charcot might well have said as he did of 'injunction,' that it is 'a remedy, the mechanism of which we know little.' We have already quoted him to the effect that 'suggestion is a difficult agent to handle; it is, if you will permit the metaphor, a drug whose accurate dosage is far from easy.'[37]

He took up Burq's methods in recognition of the principle that there were more things in heaven and earth than the natural philosophy of 1876 accounted of. In the following decade he no doubt came to know, as his utterances tell us, that whatever strikes the imagination is potentially a healing agent. He would have prescribed a bag of warm oats, had he thought it would do the patient good; on one occasion he actually did so.

The elements of saving faith cannot be summed up in as simple a word as 'suggestion,' which cloaks a multitude of psychological influences. Cure involves the strengthening of the patient's ego, the retreat of repressed mental forces, the enhancement of the patient's will to be well, and reinforcement of his desire to lead a complete and normal life. Thus, in the words of Eileen Garrett: 'The physical, mental, moral and religious atmosphere has to be taken into account, if the faith engendered is to continue to live and grow into a state of wholeness.'[38] Cures and transformations have to be regarded as responses of the deeper layers of the personality to the total psychological atmosphere. This was particularly recognized by F. W. H. Myers in the 1890's, when he rebuked the Bernheim school for their own propagandist excesses in using the blanket term 'suggestion' in too facile a way:

    . . . not one suggestion in a million reaches or influences the subliminal self. If Bernheim's theories, in their extreme form, were true, there would by this time have been no sufferers left to heal.

    . . . it must be remembered that many of the results which follow upon suggestion are of a type which no amount of willingness to follow the suggestion could induce, since they lie quite outside the voluntary realm [i.e., *conscious will*]. However disposed a man may be to believe me, however anxious to please me, one does not see how that should enable him, for instance, to govern the morbidly-secreting cells in an eruption of erysipelas. He already fruitlessly wishes them to stop their inflammation. . . .

    . . . suggestion from without must for the most part resolve itself into suggestion from within . . . the hypnotiser can plainly do nothing by his word of command beyond starting a train of thought which the patient has in most cases started many times for himself . . . but why it . . . succeeds on this particular occasion, we simply do not know. We cannot predict when the result will occur; still less can we bring it about at pleasure.[39]

Which leads very naturally to a modern formulation by Emilio Servadio: 'But what is suggestion if not a—*mainly unconscious*—search for, and acceptance of, something or someone that acts powerfully on a problem that is inside us and yet unaccessible to us?'[40]

'*Something* or *someone*,' says Dr Servadio. A magnet if it 'struck the imagination' might do, as the young man at the Salpêtrière thought at one time. But the *someone* must have been important. Though they would have indignantly denied the role of faith healers (less tolerantly, no doubt, than Charcot himself), the physicians' own personalities and intimacy with the patients, were part of the cure, and, a vital element in the total psychological atmosphere. As Eileen Garrett points out,

    One of the healer's most necessary functions . . . is to be on hand to reassure the patient : this, too, is most important in the case of the 'miraculous' cure. I have talked to many people who professed to be momentarily healed—and then found they had slipped back, because there was no reassuring voice or presence to occasionally help sustain them.[41]

Janet, in the lectures written at the Salpêtrière, makes several interesting comments on the part played by the physician in the cosmos of the patient :

> You know those patients who come to you every morning with an arm or leg contractured, asking you to 'undo that' for them. There is hardly anything to undo, but this trifle they will never be able to correct alone. . . .
>
> All those who have had to do with hystericals have also soon noticed . . . their extraordinary attachment to their physician. The doctor who attends them is no longer an ordinary man. He assumes a preponderating position, against which no other influence can prevail. For him they will do everything; for they have once for all made up their mind to obey him blindly; they think of him all the time and regulate their whole conduct after that thought. But in return they are extremely exacting; they claim him altogether, are jealous of his interest in others, make constant calls upon him, want him to stay with them, and take it really to heart if he shows the least indifference.[42]

What Janet is describing would seem almost to have the hall-marks of the psychoanalytical *transference*.

Before leaving the subject of aesthesiogenic agents, it is worth noticing that although Charcot at the end of his career probably had little faith in their special physical qualities, two ideas of Burq's seem to have had particular influence on him. Charcot's words, 'whatever forcibly strikes the mind, whatever strongly impresses the imagination,' seem to echo Burq's phrase concerning the efficacy of anything which 'strikes the imagination.' In addition, Burq attached cardinal importance to the anesthesias as the symptoms of greatest significance. To attempt the cure specifically of anesthesia was, in Burq's view, the most fundamental approach to treatment because it attacked hysteria at the root. Both Charcot's therapist Gilles de la Tourette and the Master himself seem to have adhered to this view even when Burq's methods had been long forgotten. The former regarded the reestablishment of lost sensibilities as the foundation of therapy, and the latter declared in 1891 that the hysteric is not fully cured until every trace of anesthesia has disappeared.

Chapter vii

Hypnotism Before Charcot

HYPNOTISM CAME to the Salpêtrière semiofficially about 1878, almost concurrently with metallotherapy. But the history of hypnotism had opened more than a century earlier with Franz Anton Mesmer. To say that hypnotism was totally unknown before Mesmer would be risky. Yet, the customary inferences from Egyptian papyri, suppositions about Aesculapian practice, and deductions from classical references to the 'Druid sleep' seem at best frail. All modern hypnotism stems from Mesmer.

Mesmer's theoretical ideas were drawn from a tradition with a fairly well defined line of descent from Paracelsus, who in the early sixteenth century elaborated further the old astrological theories of sidereal influence on the human personality and combined these notions with a vitalistic kind of hypothesis concerning biochemistry. In Paracelsus' system the body was endowed with a twofold 'magnetism.' One component of this magnetic force was nourished by the celestial bodies and was the source of wisdom, thought, and sensory capability. The second component was the vital principle that organized the chemical elements into living matter. According to Paracelsus there resides in each individual human being a force or power resembling that of the lodestone or electrified amber. The magnetic virtue resident in healthy persons attracts the enfeebled magnetism of the ailing. Throughout the sixteenth and seventeenth centuries, similar ideas were given currency by a succession of speculative writers, including the celebrated philosophical alchemist Robert Fludd and the van Helmonts. But great importance must be given to the Scottish physician William Maxwell writing in 1679, who regarded all diseases as resulting from a defect of a vital fluid. According to him, healing could be accomplished by restoring a requisite quantity of magnetic force. Mesmer's twenty-seven propositions promulgated in 1779 closely resemble Maxwell's exposition.

The name of van Helmont occurring in the phylogeny of mesmerism suggests for consideration yet another component source of Mesmer's methods. Van Helmont was associated with the English circle of Lady Conway, who was acquainted also with Valentine Greatrakes—'the mirabilian stroker.' Greatrakes was a celebrated Irishman who cured without fee by prayer coupled with passes of the hands—'stroking.' This is interesting, as it suggests that the mesmeric 'passes' may go back to an older tradition, a time-honored thaumaturgic practice, which perhaps has been bequeathed to modern 'spiritual healers' independently of mesmerism.

Be that as it may, Mesmer, a gamekeeper's son born near Lake Constance, graduated at Vienna in 1766, presenting a thesis *De planetarum influxu (The Influence of the Planets on the Cure of Diseases)* which attracted some attention. He described planetary influence as exerted via a subtle universal fluid with quasimagnetic powers exerted chiefly upon living matter. This 'fluid of animal magnetism' existed in two opposite forms analogous to the two types of pole in mineral magnetism, and it tended to segregate in the left and right sides of the body. The cure of diseases consisted in the restoration of disturbed balance or *harmony* between the two fluids. For some years Mesmer worked in Vienna as a physician in general practice, but he was fortunate to make a wealthy and distinguished marriage to the widow of an imperial privy councillor. This brought him into contact with the Austrian Court Astronomer, Maximilian Hell, a Jesuit Father who was interested in Paracelsian type theories and was a magnetotherapist. Mesmer assisted in treatments with magnetized 'tractors,' iron plates attached to the patients, but he soon launched into his own experiments. He replaced the magnet and traction by his own system including the fixed gaze and 'passes.' He scored some notable successes, curing his wife's companion, Fräulein Gesterlin, of a massive hysteria comprising hysterical faints, somnambulistic trances, and—interestingly enough—that rare symptom, hysterical ischuria. Mesmer soon became celebrated, but he fell foul of the fact that in the field of neurosis cures are not always appreciated. He cured the daughter of a court secretary of hysterical blindness. But the symptom returned presumably reinstituted by the same emotions that had caused the original illness. It is said that a disability pension drawn by the invalid had something to do with the attitude of Fräulein Paradis's parents. Be that as it may, they became the focus of an agitation against Mesmer in which perhaps the honest doubts and also the professional prejudices and jealousy of his medical colleagues played a part. In the event he was expelled from the medical faculty and betook himself to the intellectual capital of the world.

Paris in 1778 was receptive to new and exciting ideas. Savants such as Benjamin Franklin had heightened interest in the scope and utility of natural forces and had 'rendered the marvelous probable.'[1] Mesmer's ideas deeply impressed Charles d'Eslon, physician to the Comte d'Artois, younger brother of the King. Since d'Eslon was a leading physician of the Faculty, Mesmer had the best possible introduction to Parisian society as well as to Parisian medical circles. When his first clinic at the Place Vendôme proved inadequate, he and d'Eslon set up a larger one in the Rue Montmartre. Everyone wanted to be magnetized, and Mesmer had to employ assistants—*valets toucheurs*—to magnetize in his place. This not sufficing, he had to invent the famous *baquet*, a circular oaken trough whose floor was covered by powdered glass and iron filings. Iron rods conducted the magnetism to the hands of the patients who were arranged in several concentric circles around the *baquet*. Listening to music, they awaited the effects, often dramatic, of the magnetism. Mesmer, in a coat of lilac silk and carrying an iron wand, would walk among the patients, accompanied by d'Eslon and assistants chosen for their youth and comeliness. He would touch the bodies of the patients with the wand, or 'magnetize' them with his eyes, fixing his gaze on theirs. He would lay his hand on the affected part of the body, or make use of the famous 'passes.' Seated opposite the patient foot against foot, knee against knee, Mesmer would erect his fingers in a pyramid, pass his hands all over the patient's body, beginning with the head and going down the shoulders to the feet. He then returned again to the head, the abdomen, and the back. The process was repeated until the subject was 'saturated with the magnetic fluid' and was transported with pain or pleasure. Like the ladies at Saint Médard who called for *le secours*, young women at the Hôtel Bullion were much gratified by the *crisis* (as it was called) and begged to be thrown into it anew; they followed Mesmer through the hall and confessed that it was impossible not to be warmly attached to the magnetizer's person.[2] No doubt, the pressure of Mesmer's hands on the 'hypochondriac region' (i.e., the abdominal or ovarian area) was a specially potent factor in induction of the crisis, as formerly at Saint Médard and later at the Salpêtrière.

The crisis was, in fact, the essential stage in the cure and was recognized as such by Mesmer and the later magnetizers. It was an emotional upheaval which, as in the case of Despine's, Janet's and Sollier's patients when treated aesthesiogenically resulted in a transformation with temporary or permanent disappearance of neurotic symptoms. The emotional response of the subjects to Mesmer himself parallels the 'transference' relation between patient and physician which has already been spoken of. Indeed, it is worth continuing the quotation from Janet when speaking (in his Salpêtrière lectures) of the attachment of the neurotic patient to his doctor.

This attachment, which develops according to the treatment they require, reaches extraordinary proportions if somnambulism and suggestion become part of it. The old magnetizers, who had often, though without knowing it, hystericals in charge, noticed it, and have repeatedly described this phenomenon. Perhaps we might, in honour of the heroic period of magnetism, call it the magnetic passion. . . . He would, indeed, be a very superficial and coarse observer who would consider this passion from an erotic standpoint. . . . Hystericals, of course, may, like everybody else, have their own feelings of this kind : besides, there are not so many ways of expressing an attachment for another person, especially if that person be of the other sex. Certain subjects transform their attachment into a filial sentiment, into one of respect, of superstitious terror, or even into a maternal sentiment. . . . Truly it [the magnetic passion] may exist without being accompanied by any [of these sentiments]. An hysterical, a man of thirty, whom we had cured of a very troublesome tic, would not leave us any more, and came to see us on the slightest pretext, without having for us any kind of affection and without understanding himself why he wanted to see us. We have seen hystericals who had simultaneously a really erotic passion for one individual and a magnetic passion for another, and, without confusion, be equally engaged in rendezvous with the first and séances with the second.[3]

The 'magnetic passion' viewed somewhat superficially and coarsely (to use Janet's phrase) came under consideration in a secret appendix to the report of the Commission set up by the government in 1784 to investigate the existence of the 'magnetic fluid' whose reality was asserted by Mesmer and d'Eslon.[4] The Commission, which had been established as a result of much contention, comprised members of the Academy of Sciences and of the Faculty of Medicine. It was led by the astronomer Bailly, and among its nine members were Benjamin Franklin, Lavoisier, and Dr Guillotin. It reported that the 'animal magnetic fluid' did not exist, and that the violent effects observed in patients under public treatment were due 'to contact, to the excitement of the imagination, and to mechanical imitation of others. All public treatments by magnetism must in the end be productive of evil results.' A similar condemnation was issued simultaneously by the Royal Society of Medicine. Mesmer left France, and the first chapter in the history of animal magnetism was closed.

But Mesmer, though his discoveries were to be officially despised, left a potent legacy in France. Societies of Harmony had been formed in Paris, Strasbourg, Lyons, Bordeaux, and elsewhere. At the very moment when mesmerism was condemned in Paris, it was taking a new turn on the country estate of the estimable Marquis Armand Jacques Marc Chastenet de Puységur, who set himself to relieve human suffering by use of mesmerism. Trying to induce the crisis in Victor, a young shepherd with a chest infection, the Marquis instead found that Victor had gone into a state of 'lucid slumber,' that is, hypnotic somnambulism—essentially the 'complete somnambulism' previously discussed. In this state Victor had all his usual faculties and more; indeed, he seemed much more intelligent. Obedient to all of de Puységur's commands while in the lucid trance, Victor showed retrospective amnesia when restored to the normal waking state. De Puységur's discovery shifted the aim of the magnetizers from 'cure by crisis' to 'cure by somnambulism.'

The lucid somnambulist was supposed not only to have his normal intellectual powers and sensory perceptiveness augmented, but also, on the analogy of the prophets and sibyls of old, was believed to have supernormal abilities of clairvoyance and precognition. In fairness to the magnetizers, there is some reason to believe that on occasion the somnambulists may have exhibited abilities in the way of extrasensory perception. As a history of mesmerism and paranormal phenomena is available, this need not concern us here.[5] What is important is the impetus artificial somnambulism gave to the study of animal magnetism through all France. In addition to the existing Societies of Harmony, Magnetic Societies were formed in Paris and at Rennes, Troyes, Caen, and Rheims. In the period between 1813 when Deleuze produced his history of animal magnetism and 1850, a remarkable number of investigators engaged in the study of lucid somnambulism. These were quite different from the stage mesmerists who flourished independently of them, and from quacks and charlatans whose interest was purely commercial and who would certainly have been operative. The list of highly respectable medical men and physiologists who worked at artificial somnambulism is a long one and includes such names as Charpignon, Morin, Baron Du Potet de Sennevoy, Lafontaine, Charles Despine, and Dr Perrier of Caen—a name that later we shall find very significant. The aim of the magnetizers was to produce cures à la Mesmer, but as time went on they devoted major effort to the development of lucid somnambulists. If a patient could be brought into the somnambulist state, it was thought, he could, through the supernormal perception conferred by 'ultralucidity,' diagnose his own condition and prescribe the appropriate treatment. Even better, he could apply clairvoyant perception to diagnose the ailments of other nonlucid patients and prescribe for them. Mostly the prescriptions were absurd, but not always. Sometimes a diagnosis was correct and the prescription worked. To explain these successes we have a choice. Chance must have accounted for some of the successes. Also a proportion of the somnambulists may have had clairvoyant perception like certain modern 'sensitives.' Lastly, a somnambulist long engaged in medical practice of this kind might well have picked up a considerable degree of straight ordinary medical knowledge and diagnostic competence, aided by the refined power of normal observation which the narrowing and concentration of attention encourages under hypnosis.

The cultivation of somnambulist physicians lingered on remarkably late in the century. Janet in 1892 described Mlle Eugénie, whom he had met through Charles Richet:

> We set out for the country in the suburbs of Paris, where Mlle Eugénie lives in a small house . . . busy with the humble functions of housekeeper. She is a very pretty young girl of 22. She had been out all day giving consultations in a celebrated office, where she is assisted by a doctor, who signs her prescriptions. She has but just returned and is very tired, but she cannot remember what she could have been doing all day . . . but that does not trouble her, for she is in a hurry to prepare the soup for her aged parents. We get her to consent to our putting her to sleep for an instant. She is no longer in the somnambulic state than the whole scene changes. With head erect she falls at once into the professional language; she says authoritatively: 'Imagine, my dear sir, 31 consultations today . . . and some very interesting cases . . . I was quite right when I said that that lady was pregnant with twins; but her physician would not believe . . . all those physicians are but simpletons.'⁶

In Dr Powilewicz's *service*, Janet encountered a hysterical man who had drifted to Le Havre after spending time in various of the Paris hospitals. While they were examining a contracture under hypnosis, the patient became irritable and murmured, 'These provincial students do not even know that a contracture is taken off by striking the antagonistic muscles. Sir, should you like me to give you a lecture on hysterical paralysis?' As Janet remarks, in many cases the speeches made by people in the presence of a somnambulist, even more than suggestions properly so called, succeed in furnishing the patient with an education.[7]

The example of young Mlle Eugénie is interesting because it shows that long after the heyday of the magnetizers, their practice lived on, though their methods of induction of somnambulism might have changed and incorporated those of the hypnotists proper. Their practice was clandestine and highly unofficial, even though many of them were responsible members of the medical profession like Morel, the eminent alienist of Rouen. This secrecy resulted in some measure from the further official condemnation of animal magnetism in 1837. Back in 1820 it had seemed that the activity was about to enter upon an era of development within orthodox medicine. Dr Bertrand, a graduate of the École Politechnique who had qualified in medicine and had become one of the scientific editors of the *Globe* and *Le Temps*, gave some lectures on '*l'extase*' in 1820 and not long after produced his *Traité du somnambulisme*.[8] Bertrand was the true originator of the theory of suggestion and almost the first of the 'animists' as opposed to the 'fluidists'—a distinction that will be discussed later. Bertrand took little account of the subtle 'fluid of animal magnetism.' Aided by Charles Despine's case notes on somnambulism and other features of magnetism such as catalepsy, Bertrand proposed that the facts of animal magnetism were potentially capable of explanation in psychological terms by adequate study of the mental condition of the subjects. Bertrand should perhaps yield place to the Abbé Faria as the first animist and forerunner of hypnotism proper. A Portuguese Jesuit from the East Indies, Faria gave public demonstrations of magnetism in Paris in 1813. He departed entirely from Mesmer's methods. He seated the subject and commanded him imperiously to go to sleep. His booklet of 1819 hints at the animist position, but his insight did not rival Bertrand's.[9] Subsequent to Bertrand's attempt to bring mesmerism within the pale of official medicine, experiments were done in the Paris hospitals, at the Hôtel Dieu by Baron Du Potet at the invitation of Dr Husson, and by Georget and Rostan at the Salpêtrière.[10] The work was, however, terminated by order of the general council of the hospitals on the ground that patients should not be used for experiments.

But in 1825 a movement developed within the Academy of

Medicine favoring an objective examination of the claims of the magnetizers. The enquiry was proposed by one Foissac in terms unpropitious for its acceptance, for he asserted that somnambulist diagnosis functioned 'with an intuition worthy of the genius of Hippocrates.' Nonetheless, a Commission was set up under the chairmanship of Husson, which reported in 1831 affirming the existence of magnetism. Unfortunately, their report and the research on which it was based entirely stressed the paranormal or marvelous aspects of somnambulism—clairvoyant diagnosis, 'finger-tip reading,' and the like. As the experiments were faulty in design and statistical analysis, the report though favorable carried no conviction and was shelved. But discussion could not be suppressed, and in 1837 Dr Oudet drew attention to an entirely nonmystical application of 'magnetic sleep'—anesthesia in dentistry. The same year Du Potet visited England and inspired Elliotson to apply mesmerism in healing and for surgical anesthesia. It was during this period that Esdaile in India performed numerous operations under hypnosis. Had it not been overtaken by the development of chemical anesthetics (nitrous oxide in 1844, ether in 1846, chloroform in 1847), hypnosis, advancing by this route, might have had an easier passage.

In France in 1837, a young magnetizer, Berna, encouraged by the prospect of respectability which Oudet's announcement seemed to have opened up, implored the Academy of Medicine to look at the subject once again. Unfortunately, Berna repeated Foissac's error of tactics and directed attention to the alleged paranormal aspects of somnambulism. The resulting Commission, of which Dr Dubois was secretary, repeated the approach employed by the Husson Commission. The experiments that were aimed at testing paranormal phenomena were similarly faulty. More catastrophically, the Commission failed even to confirm perfectly normal phenomena such as anesthesia, and their report was markedly unfavourable; the third official condemnation of animal magnetism. It is a little strange that they should have failed to confirm the induction of anesthesia which had already been demonstrated practically by one of their members, Cloquet, who had performed a sizable operation on a 'magnetized' patient in 1829.[11] However, animal magnetism was relegated to the twilight mode of existence, already described, in which it was destined to remain for almost forty years, increasingly prone to be invaded by charlatans. Its fate can, in part, be ascribed to the conservatism of the medical profession but also to the magnetizers' unfortunate choice of the ground on which the battle was fought.

Though relegated to a scientific limbo and often derided, mesmerism yet enjoyed much lay popularity. Many of the clergy were enthusiastic in discussion of magnetism, and some even practiced it in the hope of getting revelation thereby. Lacordaire, the famous preacher, declared from the pulpit at Nôtre Dame that magnetism was the last remnant of the old prophetic power. In 1856 the Holy Roman Inquisition vetoed what it called the abuses of magnetism, which it regarded as a supernatural manifestation masquerading as the operation of physical forces. For centuries the *Abbés* and *Curés* had paced French fields with rods and pendulums divining for water, and this harmless recreation was still free from the taint of heresy. But the Inquisitors would not allow the 'fluid of animal magnetism' to be of the same innocent and physical nature as the force that bent the hazel twig. As the Inquisition was relatively impotent outside of the Papal States, only the clergy were much deterred by this. However, Spiritualism in its rise tended to assimilate magnetism to itself.

Meanwhile, in the mid-century new developments favored the transition from magnetism to hypnotism. The authors of hypnotism were basically 'animists' and not 'fluidists.' A book originally written in 1820 by General Noizet, a friend of Bertrand's, was published in 1854 and had considerable effect. Noizet did not delve very far theoretically, but he insisted that somnambulism occurred as a result of psychological factors rather than physical forces.[12] But it was a Manchester surgeon, James Braid, who must be regarded as the father of hypnotism —a word he coined from the Greek *hypnos*, sleep. Witnessing some public demonstrations by the Swiss magnetizer Lafontaine, whom he believed to be an impostor, Braid became convinced through his own researches that the magnetic sleep was a genuine phenomenon. He proved to his own satisfaction that no physical influence passed from the magnetizer to the subject. Braid's

179

conclusion was based principally on his discovery that hypnosis could often be induced merely by the subject gazing fixedly at some prescribed object, which need not necessarily be of striking appearance. Thus Braid tended to regard the hypnotic state as a purely physiological condition of the nervous system which could be induced by essentially physiological means.[13] This is really a third position distinct from either the 'animist' or the 'fluidist' one, and it had considerable influence later on the ideas the Salpêtrians brought to their study of hypnosis.

In a sense Braid devised a mechanistic physiological theory of hypnosis as a peculiar state of the nervous system which could be arrived at by purely physiological treatment of the subject. But he is classed as an animist for two reasons. First, his findings, which referred hypnosis to the state of the subject, militated against the fluidist theory of a force or substance proceeding from the mesmerizer. Second, his later work tended, like Faria's method, to establish the importance of verbal suggestions made to the subject, and this put him in the animist tradition. Many of Braid's discoveries were made independently in France by such investigators as Bertrand, Deleuze, Du Potet, and Charpignon.[14] But it was the transmission of Braid's experiences to France that drew the attention of official French medicine to hypnotism. Extracts from the numerous books published by Braid between 1843 and 1855 were reprinted in French medical journals and caused no great stir. But Dr Azam, a professor of medicine at Bordeaux, one of the cities that had possessed a Society of Harmony to propagate mesmerism, was familiar with magnetic somnambulism and had also learned from a colleague concerning *le Braidisme*. Albeit with some misgivings, he put this knowledge to use when called in 1858 to a patient known thereafter as Félida X, a young girl suffering from a massive hysteria characterized by spontaneous catalepsy, numerous pains, and anesthesias. Using Braid's methods to induce hypnosis, Dr Azam put her into the state he termed 'complete somnambulism,' with relief of symptoms together with restoration of cheerfulness and alertness. Azam reported this result in the *Archives de médicine* in 1860. About the same time, according to a report of Velpeau to the Academy of Medicine, Broca and Follin were using hypnosis for surgical anesthesia. Simultaneously, Guérineau amputated a leg under hypnosis. Professor Vulpian himself became interested, but surgical hypnosis was once again overtaken by the success of chloroform and the year 1860 saw both its rise and decline. But the ground for a future revanche was laid in France by a book on *Braidisme* by Durand de Gros, a physician who published under the name of Phillips, having been proscribed by the imperial government.

For another eighteen years hypnotism was officially abandoned to the secret magnetizers and the quacks and impresarios, who put on public performances. The prevailing attitude among savants was that scientific investigation was impossible because of the risk of fraud. It was assumed that subjects of hypnosis were mainly conscious simulators. A booklet by Demarquay and Giraud-Teulon which also appeared in 1860, although setting out the essential facts of hypnotism in an accurate, unsensational way, was ignored.

In the same year Liébeault, a general practitioner of Nancy, commenced work that was to be of immense significance, but destined to remain unknown until 1884, when Charcot had battered down the barrier of official acceptance. Nancy is not far from Strasbourg, which had had one of the largest of the provincial Societies of Harmony. Whether Liébeault learned of magnetism from such contacts we do not know, but having obtained cures of his own patients by suggestion under hypnotism, he retired from practice and set up a free clinic in a shed in his garden at Nancy. Liébeault was a remarkably good hypnotist; he was able to hypnotize some 90 per cent of his subjects. In 1866, he published a book that unfortunately sold hardly a copy. He sought, he says, to demonstrate the truth that 'the passive modes of existence' (i.e., hypnotic states) are 'the effects of a mental action,' and to acquaint his readers with the properties of hypnotic states 'from the point of view of the action of the *morale* upon the *physique*.'[15] Clearly, Liébeault was an 'animist.' His method of hypnotic induction was very modern. The subject had to concentrate his attention, thus minimizing the distractions afforded by sensory stimuli and by voluntary muscular movement. He stressed the rapport between hypnotizer and subject. Verbal suggestion completed the induction. Bramwell, visiting Liébeault, was amazed at the rapidity with which the patients in the relaxed informal milieu of the clinic succumbed after a few words from Liébault.[16]

Liébault labored in complete obscurity until 1882, when he attracted the attention of Professor Hippolyte Bernheim of Nancy by curing one of the latter's patients, a recalcitrant case of 'sciatica' from Strasbourg. Skeptical at first but urged by Dumont, the Professor of Physics, Bernheim was converted by seeing Liébault at work and thereafter attempted to hypnotize all the patients coming to his own clinic. Bernheim's colleagues Beaunis and Liégeois, respectively Professors of Physiology and Jurisprudence, interested themselves in the psychological and legal aspects of hypnosis. Bernheim claimed that hypnosis was successfully induced in 75 per cent of 5,000 patients over the period 1882–1886. From 1884 on, Liébault and Bernheim became famous in consequence of the first edition of Bernheim's book *De la suggestion dans l'état hypnotique*. But this was six years after the Salpêtrière researches had begun and one year after Charcot had made an honest medical subject of hypnotism, and it is hard to say how Bernheim's announcement would have been greeted if Charcot had not cleared the way.

Liébault's work, as transmitted to the world through Bernheim, proved decisive for the general acceptance of the 'animist' position. One experiment of his seems to have been crucial in converting him from a residual belief in the 'fluid' of the mesmerists. He had been in the habit of treating patients with 'mesmerized water,' which he found efficacious for curing a variety of apparently quite different maladies. To clear the matter up he did 'control experiments,' using ordinary unmesmerized spring water. A bottle of the water stood conspicuously in his consulting room where mothers brought their children for treatment. After examining the children, he pointed out the bottle to the parent, explaining that it was a potent remedy sure to heal them. Some time was devoted to the procedure, so as to impress the idea firmly on parent and child. As he obtained nineteen cures in twenty-six cases, he concluded that suggestion alone had been at work and had been effective in the waking state, without hypnosis.[17]

But these findings were unknown before 1884. It is hard to discover the route by which Charcot's interest in hypnotism was aroused. Guillain says Charcot was familiar with the publications of Braid, Broca and Follin, Azam, and Demarquay and Giraud-Teulon as well as with the writings of others, such as Mesnet,[18] and one of his own predecessors at the Salpêtrière—Lasègue. Charcot was a great reader and was unlikely to fail to note any medical publication. Charles Richet wrote extensively in the *Journal de l'anatomie et de la physiologie* as well as in Théodule Ribot's journal *Revue philosophique*, and this may have been an influence. On the other hand, the decisive factor could well have been the direct persuasion of his friends Broca and Vulpian, or (as Janet suggests) of Bourneville, Brissaud, Chambard, and Paul Richer.[19] Be that as it may, the fact is that Liébeault remaining yet unknown, hypnosis in 1878 was, in the official view of French medicine, at best a scientific curiosity meet only for a little speculative writing and at worst a field bedeviled by occultism, charlatanry, and scientific error. The prejudice against hypnotism must have seemed an immovable object, only to be budged by an irresistible force. Only a mighty hand could propel it out into the open arena of accepted scientific discourse.

CHAPTER VIII

Hypnotism at the Salpêtrière

IT WAS in 1877 that Charcot first announced to the Societé de Biologie that good results could be obtained by Burq's metallotherapy as well as by magnets. In 1878, Charcot presented patients cured of anesthesia and visual disturbances by the application of gold plates and described the phenomenon of 'transfer.' Methods *d'allures bizarres* could not, he said, inspire confidence at the outset, but one must judge by results.[1]

In 1869, Charles Richet had chanced to attend a demonstration by a magnetizer. However, it was only in 1873, when he became an intern at the Beaujon Hospital in Paris, that he was able to give serious attention to hypnotism, publishing his researches in 1875 in the *Journal de l'anatomie et de la physiologie*. Richet was particularly insistent on the genuineness of hypnotism, the hypnotic subject having so often been declared an impostor—a play actor—simulating the hypnotic state, and the hypnotizer correspondingly having been written off as a dupe or an accomplice. By skillful and pertinacious argument, Richet showed that the hypothesis of fraud was an extremely improbable one.

By 1877-78, thanks to his experience with metals and magnets, Charcot was disposed to consider techniques that like hypnotism might have a 'bizarre demeanor' in the eyes of his more conventional colleagues. Also Richet's polemics might well, in his view, have assimilated the problem of hypnotic subjects to that of hysterics. In the study of both, the question of simulation was all important. Lastly, Charcot was especially familiar with the work of Lasègue and was cognizant of the interest expressed in hypnosis by Broca, who was a friend of Azam's. It is often said that Charcot first announced hypnotism to the world as a reputable field of research in his application for membership of the Academy of Sciences in 1882, but this is not quite true. In 1878 he published in *Progrès Médical* a preliminary paper, 'Catalepsie et somnambulisme hystériques provoqués,' in which he described the use of Braid's method for induction of hypnotic states. The subjects were two young female patients at the Salpêtrière, whose names were given in abbreviated form as Louise 'Glaiz.' and Alphonsine 'Bar.' Without using the word 'hypnotism,' Charcot describes how *catalepsy* was induced by arranging for the subject to gaze fixedly at a bright light. The cataleptic state could be transformed to that of *lethargy* by gently closing the subject's eyelids or suddenly cutting off the light by interposition of a screen. Lethargy, said Charcot, was a different condition from *somnambulisme* or *sommeil magnétique*, but this third state could be induced by speaking in a peremptory tone to the lethargic subject.[2]

Charcot first used the term 'hypnotism' in papers appearing later the same year in the *Gazette des hôpitaux* and the *Gazette médicale de Paris*, in which he described the methods in use at the Salpêtrière, the characteristics of the three states just mentioned, and the phenomenon of *muscular hyperexcitability*. Hence it was no secret in the period of 1878-82 that Charcot was deeply interested in hypnotism, and that intensive work was being done at the Salpêtrière. Yet the subject had no official status outside Charcot's own sphere of influence. This circumstance did not deter Bourneville and Régnard from presenting many pictures of hypnotized subjects in the volumes of *L'Iconographie photographique de la Salpêtrière* which came out between 1877 and 1880.[3] Paul Richer included hypnotism in his book of 1881, while Ladame of Geneva who, like the Salpêtrians, had interested himself both in historical neuropathology and in magnetotherapy, published his own book on the 'hypnotic neurosis' in the same year.[4]

The title of Ladame's book indicates a preconception he shared with Charcot; namely that the hypnotic state is a kind of neurosis. In the sequel Charcot's reputation was to be heavily penalized in respect of this formulation, which became a ground of complaint against him. In 1865 Hack Tuke had coined a striking phrase when he described hypnotism as a kind of artificial insanity.[5] Insofar as an hypnotic state is not the spontaneous or habitual condition of mankind, but a state that has to be induced by some deliberately applied procedure, it is clearly accurate to describe it as abnormal. Hypnosis exhibits the following abnormal psychic features: the obedience or subjection to the hypnotizer, the sensory anesthesias that can be induced, and the tendency to retrospective amnesia. The hypnotic state can also be expressed in the form of induced physical signs—paralyses or cataplectic flexibility of the limbs. But, said Charcot, there is no anatomic lesion. The hypnotic state is on a footing with a neurosis which, Charcot came to maintain, is a purely mental malady. Consequently, it seemed quite logical to Charcot to describe the hypnotic state as an artificially induced neurosis or 'experimental neurosis,' as he did in his 1883 address to the Academy of Sciences. Thus far Charcot could not have been faulted. Any argument would have been purely about words, and if hypnotic subjects found it derogatory to be described as entering into a neurosis (even though an artificial one), yet another new word could have been coined.

But another factor dominated the situation at the Salpêtrière. At the beginning of these studies in 1877, when it was known that Charcot had become interested in hypnotism, several of his colleagues (whom Janet lists as Bourneville, Brissaud, Richer, Ruault, and Londe, the latter a chemist and director of the photographic laboratory at the Salpêtrière) brought to Charcot the two young women already mentioned, Louise Glaiz. and Alphonsine Bar., and a third patient by the name of Blanche Wittmann, frequently met with in the literature of the period as 'Witt.' or 'W.'[6] A sufferer from massive hysteria, Blanche had never for long been able to face the stresses of ordinary life and had tended to return to one or the other of the Paris hospitals after brief spells in the world. Long an inmate of the Salpêtrière, she was often pointed to as the prototype of the celebrated 'three stages'—lethargy, catalepsy, and somnambulism, whose characteristic details she realized with a marvelous precision.'[7] It is to be regretted that no complete biography of Witt. is available. She was the subject of a variety of experiments in hypnotic perception and behavior many of which became classics. Binet recounts a jest perpetrated by Londe on Blanche while she was in a state of hypnotic somnambulism. Showing her a photograph of donkeys ascending a hillside in the Pyrenées, he declared: 'Voici le votre portrait. Vous êtes toute nue!' 'Here is your portrait. You are completely naked.' Later, coming on the plate in the waking condition, Blanche stamped on it furiously. Her fury was similarly excited over a period of two months whenever she was shown a print of the same scene, presumably because it evoked the same hallucinatory appearance.[8]

According to Liégeois, Blanche was described by Jules Charetie as 'aux traits fins et doux, avec des yeux bleux tranquilles et bons.'[9] But the blue eyes were shortsighted, a fact that led to an interesting observation by Binet.[10] It was found early on that if a hypnotized subject is given an hallucination of an object and is then told to look through opera glasses, the imaginary object appears nearer, just as it would if it were real. But Blanche was shortsighted and had to adjust the glasses to bring the phantom object clearly into view. Compared to some of the other Salpêtrière subjects, who would passively accept rapidly varying suggestions as to the distance of an object while in a state of somnambulism, Blanche was rather intelligent. When a hallucinated bird sitting on a hallucinated tree was said by Binet to be now near, now far, now to the left, and now on the right, Blanche (unlike Binet's two other subjects, C and D) evinced lively astonishment and displayed a critical spirit, failing to understand why the bird on the tree should be close to her at one moment and far away at another. When Binet explained this phenomenon in terms of the bird flying about, Blanche was skeptical on the ground that the tree was shifting around also! Finally, still in somnambulism, she rationalized the matter by blaming her eyes as defective in assigning distance to objects. Blanche was also inclined to be contentious in the mirror experiment, in which the subject is given the hallucination of an object, say, a butterfly. A mirror being positioned behind the supposed location of the object, the subject usually 'sees' a hallucinatory reflection of the butterfly in the mirror. When told to pick up the second butterfly, Blanche would try a few times and, after striking the mirror with her hand a few times, would absolutely refuse to try further declaring, 'I cannot do it.'

The experiments with hallucinatory appearances carried out at the Salpêtrière were, of course, much the same as those executed at Nancy and elsewhere, once Charcot had made the subject respectable. An experiment of which Charcot himself was fond consisted in showing a subject one of a pack of blank cards and suggesting a hallucinatory picture upon it. The cards, which were marked on the back so as to be identifiable to the experimenter, were then shuffled. Strangely enough, the subjects could usually pick out the 'picture card,' even though it was as blank as the other cards. The explanation usually supplied by the experimenters was that the subject identified the card by unconscious response to minute identifying features. Another experiment that Charcot liked to demonstrate during his lectures derived from the discovery by Richer, Binet, and Féré that hallucinated objects can leave 'after images,' as normally perceived objects do. The subject was shown a piece of white paper, with the suggestion that it was red or green. A similar paper being substituted without suggestion, the subject would see it tinged with the complementary color, green or red.[11] We need not be concerned here with the validity of these experiments or their interpretation. It suffices to note the exciting range of new studies opened up by the arrival of hypnotism within the ambit of science.

But to return to Blanche Wittmann. In the period after 1884, the 'School of Nancy' in particular made it become very fashionable to discuss the 'Svengali' type of problem. The question at issue was the extent to which hypnotic subjects could be compelled by the hypnotist to commit acts foreign to their natural inclinations or ethics in the waking state. Numerous causes célèbres were argued in the courts and brought to the attention of jurists such as Liégeois and of experts on legal medicine such as Charcot's friend Brouardel. Magnetizers stood in the dock accused of seducing their more personable subjects. A wretched Parisian dentist, Levy, could hardly have been more unfortunate had his name been Dreyfus. Having extracted a tooth under hypnosis—in the presence of the patient's mother, who declared her back was turned—he was jailed for ten years when the girl became pregnant.[12] In other criminal cases, over a decade or so, it was submitted that theft or murder had been committed under hypnotic suggestion. As late as 1900 Madame Weiss in Algeria claimed she had attempted to poison her husband while under the hypnotic control of her lover. Even in England, which runs less to drama, Dr Kingsbury was accused of forcing a lady under hypnotism to make a will in his favor.[13] To settle this problem, hypnotic subjects at Nancy and Paris were frequently ordered to commit imaginary crimes—to steal the doctors' watches or to kill interns with rubber knives or toy pistols. It was the 'School of Nancy' which came to the more sensational conclusions. While affirming extremely vigorously that hypnotism was medically harmless, they sketched a rather lurid picture of its terrors in the hands of philanderers or of criminals who would commit their crimes by proxy through hypnotic commands to virtuous but hypnotizable subjects. A battle of the books resulted, Bernheim and Liégeois of Nancy[14] being answered by Gilles de la Tourette who presented the view of the Salpêtrière, a view often put forward by Charcot himself, who contended that in the charades acted out by the hypnotic subjects, the performers were perfectly aware that they were not executing real crimes but were play-acting. In the experience of the Salpêtrians, hypnotism did not alter the character of the subject; his inhibitions remained under hypnotism with regard to both major crimes and minor social usages. For example, Binet and Féré cite the patient at the Salpêtrière who would *tutoyer* one of the physicians when he visited the ward alone, but would observe the laws of good breeding and revert to the formal *vous* as soon as a stranger entered, even under somnambulism.

Blanche Wittmann, who was described as carrying out imaginary crimes with a dramatic flair equal to Sarah Bernhardt's, was much in demand for medicolegal demonstrations. On one occasion Charcot had invited a distinguished audience of jurists, magistrates, and specialists in forensic medicine to a demonstration in the lecture theatre at the Salpêtrière. Blanche, in a state of somnambulism, had obediently performed the most bloodthirsty tasks, 'shooting,' 'stabbing,' and 'poisoning.' The notables withdrew from a room littered with fictive corpses. The medical students who remained, being very like medical students in all times and places, then told Blanche (still in a state of somnambulism) that she was alone in the hall and should undress and take a bath. But Blanche, who had waded through blood without turning a hair, found this suggestion too infamous and came abruptly out of hypnosis with a violent hysterical attack.[16]

Sometime prior to 1888, Blanche was transferred to the service of Dumontpallier at the Hôtel-Dieu and came to the notice of Jules Janet, about the same time that Pierre Janet encountered Léonie at Le Havre. Jules Janet hypnotized Blanche and took her through the usual three 'classic' stages (i.e., catalepsy, lethargy, and somnambulism). But when she was in lethargy, instead of transferring her to the cataleptic stage by means of one of the recognized methods, Janet continued to make mesmeric 'passes,' and Blanche passed into an absolutely inert state (perhaps Gurney's 'deep state') and reawakened into a state resembling the 'complete somnambulism' of Azam and the metallotherapists. In this state, which amounted to a new personality, 'Blanche 2,' almost all the symptoms of 'Blanche 1'—anesthesias and flaccid paralyses—had disappeared.[17] Jules Janet, repeating the experiments of Azam and Sollier, was able to maintain Blanche in this ameliorated condition for long periods.

Blanche Wittmann typifies the type of subject on whom the Salpêtrière researches in hypnotism were based. Characterized by pronounced hysterical symptoms, these patients were potentially capable of both the 'transformation' achieved by the metallotherapists and the total somnambulism effected by Azam. Whether these patients had episodes of natural somnambulism —fugue states—other than somnambulistic phases in hysterical attacks, we cannot say. It is certain, however, that their psychic constitution was closely akin to that of the natural somnambulist. Charcot fully realized that he was working with material of the kind sought by the old magnetizers, the stuff of which the 'lucid somnambulists' and the diagnostic clairvoyants were made. Conversely, he believed that the magnetizers deliberately looked for good somnambulists among the hysterical, because early experience had shown hysterics to be the most promising subjects. Writing in 1892, Charcot remarked—with justice —that,

the most celebrated somnambulists since Puységur, who discovered somnambulism, have all suffered from *convulsive crises*, the hysterical nature of which is not even disputed. . . .

We have remarked (in accordance with Hack Tuke's observations) that so-called natural somnambulists generally become very good hypnotic somnambulists; but also we have very frequently remarked the so-called natural somnambulism in the antecedents of hysterical persons.[18]

Charcot believed that pronounced response to hypnotism was itself a trait akin to hysteria, that hypnotism could, therefore, be regarded as a pathological or morbid condition. For Charcot deep hypnosis was on a par with a severe hysterical symptom. Deep hypnosis has to be induced by an externally provided suggestion, while the hysterical symptom is induced by autosuggestion. But the difference thus stated appears secondary to the similarity. Also, the autosuggestion that ultimately generates the hysterical symptom is itself dependent in some degree on externally provided 'suggestions,' for example, the trauma in traumatic neurosis and the attitudes of the patient's relatives. Thus it is possible to reverse the argument and assimilate hysteria to hypnotism. As we said earlier, Charcot did just that, and imposed hysterical symptoms by hypnotic suggestion. Seen in the context of Charcot's main aim—the understanding of neurosis—and in the historical perspective of magnetism, natural and 'lucid' somnambulism, Charcot's standpoint seems less arbitrary and more reasonable than, speaking with hindsight, historians of medicine and hypnotism have regarded it.

It may seem unnecessarily tendentious of Charcot to have written as late as 1891 that he would 'define hypnotism to be an artificially produced *morbid* condition' (italics supplied).[19] But it has to be admitted that from the beginning he never claimed to express an opinion concerning hypnotism other than in regard to 'hypnotism in hystericals,' and he observed these terms of reference with the utmost consistency. Nothing is more easy to verify than the accuracy of Janet's remark that the theory of the hysterical nature of the deeper hypnotic states was not invented by Charcot and his school. All that the Salpêtrians did, said Janet, was to verify and confirm that theory in manifold ways. Janet declares also that he himself maintained the same theory in 1889, before he 'adhered to Charcot's school.' All his studies since then had strengthened his conviction of its soundness.[20] The theory that hypnotic phenomena ought to be classed among the symptoms of hysterical neurosis was, in fact, formulated in the early days of animal magnetism. Bertrand, about 1826, recommended animal magnetism as the best remedy for hysteria and declared that it was most effective and could most readily be induced in hysterical women. The Abbé Faria declared roundly that in hysterics the mesmerist merely developed an existing predisposition when he put them into *sommeil lucide*. Noizet knew that the subjects in whom he induced somnambulism were mainly neuropaths. Briquet quoted it as a fact well known that most of the 'magnetic somnambulists' were hysterical females.[21] In 1859, Despine asserted that hypnosis was an abnormal and essentially morbid condition that was obviously connected with hysteria. Since Charcot, physicians (named by Janet) having no connection with Charcot's school have independently put forward a very similar view. Charcot's decision to regard induced somnambulism as a special feature of hysteria was neither perverse nor original, but in the mainstream of the magnetizers' tradition.

Charcot did not deny the existence of minor hypnotic phenomena attainable in subjects without a strong neuropathic disposition. This he called *petit hypnotisme* (minor hypnotism), but he insisted that he left its study to others. He was concerned with *grand hypnotisme* (major hypnotism), the hypnotism to be found in a pronounced form only among actual or latent hysterics. There were strong arguments in favor of the view that success in inducing lucid somnambulism often corresponded to a latent disposition to hysteria even if the subject was not in fact suffering overtly from any nervous disease. Numerous magnetizers and medical hypnotists throughout the nineteenth century found that on occasion the induction of hypnosis generated or uncovered a hysterical state. Indeed, the *crises* at Mesmer's *baquet* were essentially hysterical attacks. Gilles de la Tourette, in a paper delivered before the Society of Legal Medicine in Paris in 1888, demonstrated how the passage of stage magnetizers through the towns of France had been followed by epidemics of hysteria. 'Our country has become the refuge of all the magnetizers, and their advertisements cover the walls of France.'[22]

It is an ironic fact that Charcot, who was so often accused of theatrical and dramatic presentations of hypnotism to too 'public' an audience, campaigned sternly against hypnotism practiced by amateurs or by stage magnetizers. In a paper published in 1887 in *La revue de l'hypnotisme*, devoted mainly to the cure by hypnotism of hysterical contracture, he referred also to 'une victime de l'hypnotisme,' a boy aged twelve years, 'Bla.,' who had just been released from the Salpêtrière cured of constantly repeated hysterical attacks.[23] He was a native of the little town of Chaumont in Champagne, where the preceding year a stage magnetizer had given a demonstration that so enthused some of the population that many of them, possessed by what Charcot dubbed *manie hypnotique active*, set to hypnotizing any willing subjects. Bla. was a subject who almost immediately became prone to violent convulsive crises. Being referred to the Salpêtrière he was cured within a few months, because for many years Charcot had been putting special emphasis on coping with nascent hysteria in the young. A little later on, Charcot drew attention to a case where a woman hypnotized at a fair had become aphasic for several months. Public displays of hypnotism have been forbidden in France since about 1900, but not until recently in England.

Having decided that hypnotism was a form of neurosis, Charcot embarked on its study in the same spirit as that in which he had tackled hysteria. As with hysteria, the perennial and crucial question was that of simulation or imposture. As with all nervous diseases, there was also the problem of definition. Even organic diseases were variable in their age on onset, their distribution, and the intensity of their symptoms. Charcot had succeeded in describing the essential forms of nervous disorders and in defining them as clinical types by finding cases in which the symptoms were most intense and clear-cut. Careful study of these definitive examples enabled definition of the type. The various imperfect, partial, and 'frustrated' examples of the disease could then be identified and diagnosed differentially. In 1878 therefore, when introducing the subject to the medical public, Charcot stressed that the studies at the Salpêtrière were limited not only to patients with *hysteria major,* but also to those subjects who exhibited the characteristics of the hypnotic state in their most developed and clear-cut form. He added that it seemed more *philosophique* (i.e., *methodologically* more scientific) to deal with the extreme and more regular cases before discussing those whose expression was more rudimentary and less distinct, that is, the *formes frustes.* Elsewhere Charcot makes it clear that even among Salpêtrière patients, reactions to hypnotism were rather varied. However, he deliberately looked for examples that, because of their close similarity, sufficed to define a type. As a result of this desired homogeneity, Salpêtrian hypnotic research was based mainly on about a dozen patients including the three originals—Bar., Glaiz., and Witt. Like the earlier magnetizers from Bertrand to Despine, Charcot's assistants found that their good subjects were all female hysterics of a pronounced kind. Thus the work at the Salpêtrière in the field of hypnotism, as a result of the traditional opinions of the medical magnetizers and as an outcome of Charcot's own mode of approach to organic nervous diseases, was made to rest on a somewhat narrow base. In later years, this situation was to lead to much criticism. In retrospect we can see it as being almost preordained in consequence of the legacy of magnetism and Charcot's own methodology.

Almost foreordained, but not quite. Charcot's sample of subjects exhibited an uncanny homogeneity of response. They all went regularly and predictably through the three phases or states—from catalepsy to lethargy, or vice versa, and then into somnambulism. In each phase the subjects presented appropriate and identical reactions to stimuli. Had the sample not been, from the start, so strikingly homogeneous, it is certain that Charcot would have realized that in hypnosis he was dealing with a very protean and variable condition, and it is likely that his line of thought would have developed differently. However, the similarity of response in his good somnambulists was an objective fact. Charcot respected facts and never failed to attempt inferences from them. Thus, his description of hypnosis turned out to be a far more rigidly systematized one than any student has subsequently dared to formulate. The homogeneity of the sample by which Charcot was misled is an interesting historical mystery for which Janet, long after, provided a solution. For the time being, we shall delay the dénouement.

Charcot was well aware of the psychological aspects of hypnotic states; he knew that psychological factors entered into the induction of hypnosis. But he regarded the psychological aspects of the problem as too subtle to be considered at the outset of the research. He therefore wished to arrive at an objective, but purely phenomenological, description of the phenomena. He thought of hypnotic states as peculiar conditions of the whole nervous system. As such they would, admittedly, be characterized by psychological peculiarities; but they were also characterized by physiological ones. The latter would be, in principle, susceptible of precise description; such a physical description ought therefore to be attempted.

Because of this bias toward the physiological (and therefore the definable and reproducible), Charcot gave preference to somewhat mechanical means of inducing hypnosis. In this he followed Braid, who had ascribed the success of his method to concentrating the attention of the subject on a fixed point until fatigue set in. Charcot also favored the method of Lasègue: Gentle pressure by the fingers on the eyeballs. Exposure to a bright light resembled Braid's method and presumably operated through induced fatigue. More dramatic methods, such as exposure to the sound of a blow on an oriental gong, seemed to operate by shock. This constituted an interesting parallel with the traumas that emerged as traumatic neuroses. Indeed, the parallel between the hypnoid state consequent on physical trauma and the hypnotic state induced by noise, bright lights, or the 'confusional technique' must have seemed very close. As a matter of fact, the analogy is pointed out both by Binet and Féré and by Janet.[24/25]

Whatever the treatment adopted, the selected subjects usually went fairly easily into the cataleptic state, in which the pulse was slackened, the breathing was superficial, and very often the subject showed complete anesthesia. Charcot and Gilles de la Tourette advised that the subject should not be kept in this state too long, lest a hysterical attack supervene. The state owed its name to the fact of catalepsy. The subject seemed totally unaware of her surroundings, or of what might be done to her. In particular, she exhibited *flexibilitas cerea* (waxen flexibility). If, for example, an arm was raised and molded into a bent position, it would remain for a considerable time in the form in which it had been placed. Now it would seem, at first sight, as if catalepsy was extremely easy to consciously simulate. But here Charcot's experience with hysteria came readily to hand; it was not for nothing that the Professor kept two pins for testing anesthesia in a pincushion on his office desk. Similarly, the muscular tremor and breathing of the cataleptic hypnotized subject holding out her arm could be followed in exactly the same way as in the hysteric whose arm was maintained in contracture. Unlike the normal person in the waking state who showed disturbed breathing and tremor if he held his arm out too long, the hypnotized hysteric with an arm in a cataleptic position showed neither of these objective signs of distress, but resembled the waking hysteric with a spontaneous contracture.[25]

The cataleptic subject could easily be put into lethargy, a state of complete relaxation, inattention, and anesthesia, yet characterized by a peculiar muscular reactivity to certain stimuli. A gentle pressure on a muscle would cause that muscle immediately to contract; the same effect would result from a light tap. Pressure on a superficial motor nerve would similarly determine the contraction of the muscles it normally activates. The muscular contractions persisted, the limb being maintained in the corresponding contracture. To undo the contracture, however, a similar stimulus applied to the antagonistic muscles would suffice. Charcot christened this responsiveness of the muscles to light stimuli during the lethargic state 'neuromuscular hyperexcitability.' A similar response, in more muted form, had already been recognized in some hysterics in the waking state. The tendon reflexes, muted in organic disease, were sometimes exaggerated in hysterics. An hysterical contracture could sometimes be induced in a limb by tight bandaging or by pressing or kneading the muscles. Thus Charcot thought that under hypnosis he had a way of studying inherent tendencies of the hysterical constitution—tendencies that hypnosis displayed in a more emphatic form.

The subject could be brought into somnambulism from either the cataleptic or the lethargic state by a variety of methods.

Somewhat curiously (and Charcot agreed that it was curious) it was possible to make the transition by rubbing the top of the subject's head lightly with the fingers or the palm of the hand. Neuromuscular hyperexcitability was still exhibited in the somnambulist condition and could be produced by very light friction.

The immediate result of Charcot's investigations of the physical signs of hypnosis was to exempt hypnotized subjects from the charge of fraud. Another possible line of defence against the foes of hypnosis was the production of blisters on the skin of subjects by giving them appropriate suggestions under hypnotism, because objective signs of this sort could not be easily simulated. Charcot, before Bernheim did so, described the appearance of pemphigoid vesicles on the arm of a hysteric some hours after the patient had received this suggestion while in somnambulism. But Charcot gave less weight to results of this sort, which were more capricious and unrepeatable than the anesthetic and muscular reactions already described.

Such was the impetus given by Charcot to *hypnosis redivivus*, as Hack Tuke called it, that numerous papers on hypnotism appeared in learned journals from 1880 until 1882. In 1883, a vacancy occured in the *Académie des Sciences de l'Institut de France*, the nation's loftiest scientific body. Interestingly enough, this vacancy arose from the demise of the aged Professor Cloquet, who had performed an amputation on a hypnotized patient in 1829 and had signed the Dubois Report opposing magnetism in 1837. Charcot was nominated a candidate for election. In earlier days as we have already mentioned, he had not had such easy success in winning academic honors as some of his contemporaries, for example, Vulpian, who became *Professeur de la Chaire* before Charcot. When a candidate in 1860 for membership of the Agrégation (i.e., attainment of the grade of faculty member, *Professeur Agrégé*), Charcot had almost failed for diffidence and nervousness. The Faculty retained a peculiarly medieval form of examination in which the applicant had to deliver an address to a tribunal of professors as well as submit a written thesis. Charcot's thesis on 'Chronic Pneumonias' was sound enough, as was his address on 'Intestinal Hemorrhages.' But he hurried through his speech nervously, feeling that his delivery was poor. Filled with a sense of failure he would have left the room if Rayer, who was on the tribunal, had not —with a commanding gesture—insisted that he stay.[26]

Consequently, in presenting his claim for election to the Academy of Sciences, Charcot might have been expected to play it safe and to submit only papers that were as orthodox and uncontroversial as possible. For instance, he could have emphasized his great work on cerebral localization which appeared that same year. However, in his *Exposé de titres et travaux* he gave pride of place to the investigations on hypnotism. He was at great pains to separate the scientific approach, as employed at the Salpêtrière, from the occultist and uncritical enthusiasm of the devotees of animal magnetism :

> a prudent and conservative orientation was developed and applied to these investigations. This approach was only slightly influenced by the purely arbitrary skepticism practised by those who, under the pretext of 'purely scientific orientation,' concealed a prejudice to see nothing and to hear nothing. . . . At the same time every attempt was made to avoid being attracted by the esoteric or the extraordinary, a peril which in this scientifically unexplored field was encountered, so to speak, at every step of the way.[27]

The method adopted, said Charcot, avoided 'pursuit of the unexpected and the mystic' and attempted 'to analyze the meaning of the clinical signs and physiological characteristics that can be identified among various conditions and phenomena caused by nervous reactions.' The study, he said, was restricted to the simplest and most constant factors and reserved to a later stage the more complex or evasive phenomena. Moreover, the study proposed to omit 'those phenomena which are of a more obscure nature and which for the moment do not appear to correlate with any known physiological mechanisms.'

On the day of the election an article signed 'Ignotus' appeared in *Figaro*, attacking Charcot for studying hypnotism and demonstrating hypnotized patients at his lectures. (Axel Munthe claims that Charcot, angered thereby, believed that Munthe had supplied information for the article. But Munthe's memory does not seem to be trustworthy in all respects, for he dates this episode in the last years of de Maupassant, who became insane in 1891 and died in 1893.)[28] Sometime later, Charcot received a pathetic letter from a paralyzed invalid requesting a medical visit. Charcot hastened to the patient who confessed that he was the Baron—(of which creation he derived his title, whether Bourbon, Orleanist, Bonapartist, or *soi-disant*, is not stated) who, under pressure of poverty, had written the scurrilous article, of which he deeply repented, at the instance of three members of Charcot's profession. 'I will treat you,' said Charcot, 'but, this time, there will be no question of any fee.'[29] As regards Charcot's temper, the impression gained from the numerous accounts of his students is that he was basically even-tempered, absorbed, and placid, with a strain of sensitivity which occasionally burst out in a flash of summer lightning, but seemed to leave little lasting resentment. The pensive forehead, and somber face, the scrutinizing eyes, the lips that bespoke silence, the impassive and impenetrable mask, like that of a Caesar (as described by Dr Souques, Charcot's last *Chéf de Clinique*)—these features gave rise to the myths of Charcot's coldness and of his tendency to adopt a pose. Yet Souques points out that the austere presence and reserved manner, the economy of words and gestures were natural to Charcot.[30]

But equally natural was the warm excitable talker, apt to jump up and down while discussing an interesting theme with those he knew and trusted, who found rapport easy with the man behind the mask. Professor Brissaud, who ran the clinical teaching at the Salpêtrière for a year after Charcot's death, testified to the non-exclusive character of Charcot's kindliness: 'Everybody here, French or foreigner, could claim the right to join the program. They were all accorded the same warm benevolence.'[31]

Brissaud referred to physicians, chemists, physiologists, philosophers, and even artists, who had received guidance, training, and inspiration 'from him who [sic] we could familiarly call "The Boss" [*Patron*] without implying disrespect.' Professor Debove recounted that, as the presiding member of a Faculty tribunal judging a thesis by one of his own students, he had spoken of the strong feelings a master has for his pupil:

I pointed out that I was in a good position to appreciate this fact, because I was seated beside my teacher Charcot. . . . Those who then could have watched Charcot from afar would have seen his face darken and assume a severe air, but I, who was next to him, saw a tear well in the corner of his eye. This exemplifies why he seemed so different to those who saw him from a distance and to those who observed him close by.[32]

Despite Ignotus' attack and the risk Charcot took of being tainted with 'magnetism,' he was elected to the Academy, receiving forty-six votes to the twelve obtained by Sappey, the other candidate. Janet remarked later that,

the Academies had already thrice condemned all researches into animal magnetism and . . . it was a signal exploit to make this learned society listen to a lengthy description of kindred phenomena. Charcot achieved this, not only thanks to his high standing in the scientific world, but also because of the method he had employed. . . . An additional point in his favour was the general trend of his paper, which presented the phenomena described as nothing more than the symptoms of a special disease. The members of the Academy, in general, like Charcot himself, believed that this study was in a field remote from animal magnetism, and was the final condemnation of the latter.[33]

Charcot's breakthrough resembled the rupture of a dam. The study of animal magnetism was now respectable under another name. The literature of magnetism suggested innumerable researches in which old discoveries could be resurrected and passed off as new. A vast literature appeared, together with new journals devoted to hypnotism. The torrent continued happily until 1884, when its direction was somewhat modified by the appearance of the first (1884) edition of Bernheim's *De la suggestion*. It is possible (though no information at all is available on this point) that Bernheim's initial interest in hypnotism, which dates from 1882, resulted in part from news from Paris. Be that as it may, Bernheim ascribed all of his knowledge of hypnotic method to Liébeault. However, he spoke of Charcot's experiments as memorable and acknowledged that it would have been impossible to overcome the prejudices against hypnotism without the prior success of Richet and Charcot. He reported cures of hysterical disorders by hypnotism (anesthesias, astasia-abasia, hysterical attacks, and mutism) just as they were effected at the Salpêtrière, but also cures by the magnet, which he still regarded as important. He reserved his opinion on the occurrence of neuro-muscular hyperexcitability, which he did not find in patients who had not been told to expect it. The germ of future controversy could be found in the stress he laid on the 'animist' interpretation; that is, that hypnosis represented primarily the results of suggestion and that, correspondingly, emphasis on hypnosis as a physiological state was perhaps misplaced. Bernheim also insisted that all the phenomena of hypnotism and suggestion could be induced in normal persons. But he spoke mostly of experiments made on hystericals and drew most of his conclusions from studies made on such subjects. Thus the divergence between the Nancy and the Parisian outlooks was not, as yet, very marked.

Meanwhile Charcot was liable to attack from a different quarter. At the Faculty lectures given in the lecture theatre on Fridays during the university term to a large audience of physicians and medical students, Charcot would demonstrate patients with a variety of organic diseases, together with hysterical patients in the waking state and under hypnosis. From the case histories quoted earlier, which are entirely typical of Charcot's procedure, it is evident that these demonstrations were perfectly decorous. All the same, Charcot has been charged with theatricality even in respect to the Friday lectures. To some extent this charge results from the fact that he was something of an innovator. In his concern to be really informative he did (as Janet said) everything possible

to attract attention and to captivate the audience by means of visual and auditory impressions. The much-discussed dramatizations of his lectures on hysteria were not at all confined to hysteria. The dramatizations were present to the same degree in his lectures on *multiple sclerosis* or on *tabes dorsalis*. The patients who were selected and presented, whether individually or in groups, whether similar or dissimilar, the schematic figures on the blackboard, the graphic résumés, the [lantern] projections, the entire show had been designed for teaching purposes.[34]

Guillain tells us that in the course of a lecture Charcot himself would often mimic clinical signs—a facial paralysis, the posture of the hand in a nerve paralysis, or the muscular rigidity of a patient with parkinsonism. The difference between the mask and the man behind it was strongly expressed at these lectures. Charcot was not a natural orator; indeed, he disliked rhetoric and pomposity. He approached the amphitheater with nervousness and timidity. Guillain quotes Charcot's former students to the effect that the *patron* spoke slowly, with impeccable diction and without gestures. 'His descriptions were always remarkably clear. He gave the impression of wanting to teach and to convince.' The lectures were devised with great care and long preparation. Written in longhand, they could have been published without correction. Yet Charcot never read from his text; he delivered the address from memory. From Freud's account of the lectures, it appears that at times the confident *patron* took over.

> As a teacher, Charcot was positively fascinating; each of his lectures was a little masterpiece in construction and composition, perfect in style, and so impressive that the words spoken resounded in one's ears and the subject demonstrated remained before one's eyes for the rest of the day.
> . . . Maître Charcot himself made a strange impression during these lectures; usually bubbling over with vivacity and cheerfulness, with witticisms always on his lips, he would appear at such moments solemn and serious, nay, even aged in his velvet cap; his voice seemed muffled, and we almost understood how malicious strangers could accuse the whole performance of theatricality.[35]

In addition to these lectures from the Professorial Chair, Charcot continued his *Leçons du Mardi*. After 1882 these changed their form, being informal clinical demonstration classes to a selected audience of Salpêtrian interns and staff, visiting physicians, old friends from the Paris hospitals, and others present by invitation. As described in Georges Guinon's paper on *La Policlinique de M. le Professeur Charcot*, about 1,900 new cases a year came to the clinic, of which about 180 were epilepsy, 200 were neurasthenia, and about 250 were hysteria.[36] Each Tuesday morning Charcot looked through the notes provided by the *Chéfs de Clinique* and selected cases that appeared to exhibit points of interest or raise problems of diagnosis. In the afternoon in a room in the outpatient clinic itself, Charcot would interview the patients, classify their symptoms, attempt diagnosis, and prescribe treatment. Discussion was free, and he would speculate more widely than in the Friday lectures. Freud wrote :

> There he examined cases quite unknown to him, risked all the chance occurrences of an interrogation, laid his authority aside and confessed at times that in one case diagnosis was impossible and that in another appearances had deceived him. Never did he appear greater to his students than on these occasions, when he thus did his best to lessen the distance between teacher and pupils by giving them a complete and faithful account of his own train of thought by stating his doubts and misgivings with the utmost frankness.[37]

As early as 1878, Charcot had included hypnosis in the topics of his Tuesday lectures. These were well attended by the medical public, including correspondents of scientific and even lay journals. The London *Times* of January 23, 1879, reprinted an extract from an article by a Dr Cartaz in *La Nature* which describes Charcot's demonstration of the three states in a patient and mentions him inducing catalepsy by sounding 'a gigantic tuning fork.' After 1882, these lectures were replaced by the Tuesday clinics. It is likely that Charcot's audiences were comprised mainly of professional medical men. Axel Munthe, writing about 1925, was very outraged that on occasions the lectures (presumably the Friday ones) were attended by lay people.[38] But this seems quite natural when we recall the association of interests in psychology that led to the foundation in 1885 of the Society of Physiological Psychology, which comprised philosophers and men of letters as well as physicians. Doubtless, members of a yet broader circle came by invitation to occasional lectures. It should be recollected that Charcot and his co-workers had wide interests. Some claim that Goncourt followed his descriptions of hysterical tics and mutism, and that traces of Charcot's influence can be found in Pirandello. Be that as it may, the 'public' character of the Salpêtrière lectures and clinics is, like the reports of Mark Twain's death, greatly exaggerated. Part of the notoriety attached to Charcot's demonstrations can be ascribed to the fact that the stage magnetizers, who now called themselves hypnotists, cashed in on the *cachet* (seal of approval) awarded to their subject by the savants and advertised their performances as 'in the style of Charcot at the Salpêtrière.'[39]

Various criticisms leveled at Charcot by the 'School of Nancy' in later years and by twentieth-century historians have, perhaps, been given more weight than is their due. It is held against him that he was somewhat reserved in regard to the therapeutic efficacy of hypnotism. But as we have seen, hypnotism for treatment was tried extensively at the Salpêtrière. Charcot himself made the modest statement that 'Hypnotism may be of some service, but not so much as one might *a priori* expect; it may be employed against some local syptoms.'[40] This opinion was indeed quite well based, being founded on several incontrovertible facts. As with other modes of therapy with hysterics, success in curing one symptom is frequently followed by its substitution with another. Again, success may only be temporary. Although in these days hypnotherapeutics have come into their own, it is still true that relapses occur in a moderately high proportion of cases. Such failure is, of course, a feature of all psychological healing, even in the religious sphere. Charcot was fond of telling the story of a young doctor who cured a patient of hysterical mutism by hypnotic suggestion. She relapsed a week later and was cured again. But the periods of remission became ever shorter, until the physician had to hypnotize her at two-hour intervals; at which he gave up, and brought her to Charcot.[41] A further problem encountered at the Salpêtrière was that not all patients were hypnotizable. Freud's experience in this connexion is worth a mention. He visited Liébeault at Nancy in 1880 and, on returning to Vienna, started to hypnotize his own patients. He said there was something positively seductive in hypnotism which gave him a sense of overcoming his helplessness. Also, it was highly flattering to enjoy the reputation of a miracle worker. In time, however, Freud found that he could not put individual patients into as deep a state as he wished, and many were completely unhypnotizable. This was not entirely due to his faulty technique, for even Bernheim had failed to cure one of Freud's patients and had admitted to Freud that his greatest therapeutic successes were achieved only with hospital patients, never in his private practice. Freud soon went over to the cathartic method of healing by the release of traumatic memories under hypnosis—Breuer's discovery. Why Freud finally abandoned hypnotism is an oft told tale. While one of his patients was undergoing the cathartic treatment, on waking she suddenly embraced Freud. He says that he had now grasped 'the mysterious element that was at work behind hypnotism.'[42] This is not the place to discuss psychoanalytic theories of 'transference.' It suffices to note that Freud had unwittingly encouraged the 'magnetic passion' of the old mesmerists.

Charcot had also been censured for stressing that hypnotism could be dangerous except in very skilled hands, because it can uncover hysterias or somnambulisms. But this, of course, was an entirely factual statement. Charcot, who campaigned against stage hypnotists, merely said that the practice of hypnotism should be restricted to medical men experienced in the field. Contrariwise, he was also attacked for underestimating the dangers of hypnotism as used in his own bailiwick, the Salpêtrière. Babinski, after Charcot's death, thought that the hypnotically induced 'symptoms,' such as paralyses and contractures, tended to endure. But Janet disagreed and thought that Babinski exaggerated.[43] Charcot himself was rather cautious. While in lectures he would reassure a class that what suggestion could do it could undo, on occasion he would say of an induced paralysis: 'Gentlemen, I dare not prolong this experiment overmuch.' A comparatively small number of patients, massively hysterical women like Blanche Wittmann, were certainly hypnotized repeatedly for purposes of research and demonstration. In this respect the Salpêtrière was no better and no worse than Nancy and many other centers. Axel Munthe attacked the hospital bitterly in retrospect, though he himself had been one of the offenders, visiting the Salpêtrière to experiment in telepathy with 'one of these girls, one of the best somnambulists I have ever met.' Writing much later, he claimed that the girls spent their days in 'semi-trance' and were consequently headed for insanity.[44] As they were almost certainly already natural somnambulists or extreme hysterics, it is unlikely that these girls would have been seriously worse off under hypnotic suggestion; nor would insanity have been the outcome. Still, we can agree with Janet's moderate verdict that the situation in which these women were involved during the early and doubtless over-enthusiastic years, if not dangerous, cannot be regarded as entirely wholesome. The balance of injury and benefit from hypnotism in the case of these young women is a fine one and is open to much discussion (see Janet). Axel Munthe was finally expelled from the Salpêtrière by Charcot for a wildcat scheme in which, using hypnosis, he tried to 'rescue' one of these patients, a pretty young girl from Normandy. Axel's son, Gustaf Munthe, attempts no defense of his father's aberration, but says that despite this contretemps, Charcot was a decisive and positive influence on Axel's development as a physician.[45]

In 1886 Bernheim published a second edition of his book on suggestion, in which he made a definite attack on Charcot's teaching. In part this may have been provoked not by Charcot himself, who did not add to what he had already said, but by some of his pupils who had been rash enough to attack Bernheim as unscientific because he did not recognize the three classic phases as found in the Salpêtrian patients. Also, some of the Salpêtrian adherents in the Paris hospitals, for example, Dr Luys at Charité, had written uncritical descriptions of their exploits in achieving transfer by magnet of symptoms from one patient to another, and so forth. Skepticism as to the physiological assumptions made in Paris was, therefore, justifiable. Bernheim announced that the three phases could be produced at Nancy, as well as the more *outré* phenomena, but only if the kind of result desired was conveyed to the subject by suggestion, direct or indirect. Bernheim also declared that all individuals were hypnotizable, though in varying degree. For the year 1880, he gave the following figures of depth of hypnotism attained in 1,014 subjects:

Unhypnotized	....	27
'Somnolent'	....	33
Light 'sleep'	....	100
Deep 'sleep'	....	460
Very deep 'sleep'	....	232
Light somnambulism	...	31
Deep somnambulism	......	131

Sex and age of subject had but minor influence.[46]

Charcot said little in public. Occasionally he said he did not wish to debate about words. *His* studies were on hypnotism in hysterics. 'Minor hypnotism' was, no doubt, interesting and a proper field of research, but it was not what he had studied. Some of his students and followers were less discreet. However, by the time Charcot died, Nancy had effectively won the battle despite some countersuccesses by Paris in the matter of criminal suggestions to hypnotics. After Charcot's death his students gave up the fight. Some of the medical profession saw with regret the decline of the Salpêtrian doctrine that had been appealingly simple and clear-cut : hypnotism was an expression of a peculiar state of the nervous system, and was characterized by definite physical signs that could be studied in an objective way by the ordinary methods of pathology. But to others Bernheim's thesis, which was the 'animist' one, had its own attractive simplicity of a different order : Hypnosis was a 'normal' phenomenon and a psychological one, induced and regulated entirely by 'suggestion.' Of course, this viewpoint had its weaknesses too. It could be pointed out that it was too simple. 'Suggestion' was an unanalyzed term, concealing a complex reality. It could justly be said that 'suggestion' was invoked as an undefined entity as universal and mysterious as the 'odylic force' or 'fluid' of the magnetists. Similarly, it could very pertinently be asked why different individuals attained such different depths of hypnosis. Indeed these questions are still with us!

However, *la suggestion* was taken to the bosom of the medical public, and 'suggestive therapeutics' blossomed luxuriantly throughout France and elsewhere. Hypnotic treatment and cure by verbal suggestion without hypnosis both became fashionable, which merely exemplified Charcot's dictum that suggestion may be quite as effective without hypnotism as in the hypnotic state. Successes obtained by suggestion, with or without hypnotism, were of course restricted largely to neurotic conditions.[47]

For about a decade after Charcot's death hypnotism flourished. Then it underwent a strange decline. It is difficult to suppose that the quarrel between Nancy and Paris was responsible, though this is often cited as the reason, because the triumph of Bernheim was so complete. Old prejudices, similar to those deployed against the magnetizers, rose again.[48] Another factor may be found in the generality and simplicity of Bernheim's teaching, which on examination seemed to have little of 'scientist's science' in it. Moreover, it transferred hypnosis into the realm of psychology, which many physicians felt to be an insecure domain into which they were not qualified to penetrate. Yet another cause may perhaps be found in the long-standing association between hypnosis and the 'supernatural'—telepathy and clairvoyance—which had continued as a theme of research through the period of Charcot and Bernheim. Whatever the reasons, hypnosis declined once more into a long twilight from which it was finally delivered only by the exigencies of medical treatment in World War II. Even the victorious Bernheim deserted hypnotism early. Suggestion soon followed hypnotism. In 1901, Bernheim admitted to a lack of precision in the use of the term 'suggestion,' and the era of 'persuasion' or 'philosophical healing' came in, about the same time as psychoanalysis was making its way in the world. Even the *Revue d'hypnotisme* changed its name in 1910.

The blame for the decline of hypnotism is today usually placed on the broad shoulders of either Freud or Charcot. The truth is doubtless more complex than that. It is still interesting, however, to consider the prime reason for the failure of Charcot's system. It fell because the majority of other workers did not confirm the occurrence of the three phases : more precisely—catalepsy, lethargy, neuromuscular hyperexcitability, and the transition to somnambulism by friction on the vertex. It is usually said that the three phases with their characteristic 'symptoms' were an artefact peculiar to the Salpêtrière. When it became necessary to explain why this artefact and no other was found there, resort was sometimes had to the same explanation as that used (prior to Charcot) for hysteria; namely, voluntary simulation or imposture by the patients. But this explanation overlooked the Charcot checks of anesthesia and muscular fatigue. Babinski, too, looked into this matter. He tried to get confessions from discharged patients long after they had left the hospital, but the results were always negative.[49] Salpêtrian hypnotism must thus be inferred to be the result of 'training' by suggestion, either direct or indirect.

But why did Salpêtrian hypnotism take its precise form? Was it invented by Charcot, or by Broca or Bourneville? Now it was and is often enough stated, with the total confidence that is apt to proceed from complete ignorance of the history of a subject, that Charcot's characteristic hypnotic phenomena were never seen outside the Salpêtrière. Yet Heidenhain in Germany and Tamburini and Seppili in Italy observed neuromuscular hyperexcitability, and the latter pair of authors obtained the three phases in their patients, though Tamburini preferred to regard some of the 'symptoms' as characteristic of hysteria rather than hypnosis. Other investigators found the states in somewhat modified or 'hybrid' form. These observers included Pitres, Dumontpallier, Magnin, and Bottey. More significant, three phases of hypnotism bearing a close, if imperfect, resemblance to catalepsy, lethargy, and somnambulism are to be found in the writings of a whole series of medical magnetizers starting with Pététin (1787) and followed later by Despine (1840), Teste (1845), Baragnon (1853), and Hébert de Garnay (1855). Puel in 1855 described paralysis induced in catalepsy by friction on the muscles. Du Potet in his *Manuel* had the three phases and recommended rubbing the head to get transitions between states.[50] Accordingly, it is clear that Charcot's hypnotism, which he believed would discredit animal magnetism, derived in fact from the old magnetizers.

We owe this discovery to Janet, who pointed out that the medical magnetizers were worthy men devoted not to the pursuit of gold, or fame, or even of knowledge for its own sake. Instead, they labored to find and train the lucid somnambulist, whose clairvoyant perception would heal the ills of his fellow men. Their problem was not easy, says Janet :

The question was, how to produce, experimentally and at the desired moment, an extensive psychological modification; and how to restore the subject to the normal state without much trouble . . .

Those who are hardy enough to attempt the solution of such a problem must perforce study the mental condition of their subjects, . . . to recognize the somnambulist modification whenever it occurs.[51]

The medical magnetizers were obliged to be keen and patient psychological observers, recording in detail every fact about the subject and every occurrence during the hypnotic sitting.

Janet stumbled on these truths and obtained the casenotes of one of the medical magnetizers while working at Le Havre with Léonie, who had previously been hypnotized by Dr Gibert. Janet himself had never before encountered the three phases. Thus he was very surprised to find something very similar to them in Léonie. There was nothing in his experience with other subjects to suggest that he had inadvertently implanted these responses in Léonie; nor could he ascribe Léonie's training to Gibert. Investigation disclosed that Léonie had a strange and eventful life story. A sleepwalker in childhood and later a hysteric, Léonie as a native of Caen, where magnetism had flourished, came to the notice of local medical magnetizers. Trained as a clairvoyant somnambulist, she had been employed as a treasure seeker as described in a little book by De Baïssas— Les trésors du Château de Crèvecœur (1867). Next she was studied carefully by Dr Perrier of Caen and at one time was 'magnetized' by Du Potet himself. In 1884, when Janet encountered Léonie, Perrier was dead, but his son provided Janet with his casenotes, exhaustive and detailed, as was to be expected from a medical magnetizer. From these records and from Perrier's published writings it was clear that Perrier's subjects exhibited the three phases, cataleptic postures and reflex hyperexcitability. Léonie's responses in 1884 were relics of 'somnambulic exercises' she had carried out as Perrier's subject in 1860.

Interestingly enough Pierre Janet, using the same method as that employed by his brother Jules with Blanche Wittmann (and doubtless recommended to Jules by Pierre), succeeded in effecting a 'transformation' of Léonie's personality very similar to that already described in the case of Blanche.[52] The original subjects Witt., Bar., and Glaiz. brought to Charcot in 1878 were thus cut from the same cloth as had interested the old magnetizers. But a further historical link with animal magnetism has to be postulated. According to Pierre Janet, this connection is not hard to find. Long before Charcot's day Husson, Du Potet, and many others had carried out experiments up and down the clinics of the Paris hospitals. A not inconsiderable number of physicians at some stage in their career had attended Du Potet's lectures at the Palais Royal. When Charcot decided to interest himself in hypnotism, a leading exponent of magnetism—the Marquis de Puyfontaine—was available, and what was more natural than for Charcot's students and collaborators to call in the expert to train the subjects and to show how it should be done? The Marquis was therefore brought to *le service de M. le Professeur Charcot*, and the preliminary experiments were carried out under his guidance.

> The experimenters wanted to . . . show Charcot the most characteristic phenomena . . . the ones that would be most striking to a man accustomed to precise neurological observations. Certain changes of state, certain simple and interesting reactions, were induced again and again in the subjects by persons who were quite unaware that they were drilling their patients.[53]

By the time Janet came to the Salpêtrière, Charcot probably knew the truth, that despite his neurologist's methodology he had fallen under the long shadow of the magnetizers. It may be, as Guillain suggests, that Charcot would have modified his theory of hypnosis as part of his revision of his ideas on hysteria. But in 1891, Charcot became a sick man whose days were numbered. Else he might have added his own postscript to one of the most curious episodes in scientific history.

CHAPTER IX

Charcot and the Supernatural

THE HISTORICAL enquiries Charcot encouraged illuminated many dark corners of human experience. Phenomena of religious fervor and of supposed demonic possession were placed in a correct medical and psychological perspective. The *Bibliothèque Diabolique* (see the Appendix) contains much that has not yet been superseded by more recent scholarship. The case of Françoise Fontaine is a document whose interest is hard to exhaust, and it still holds an important place in the critical study of those enigmatic happenings—physical mediumship and 'poltergeist' phenomena.[1] De Moray's Introduction to the *Procès Verbal de Françoise Fontaine* draws extensively on observations made in the hysterical wards of the Salpêtrière and explains some of the obscurer aspects of the witch tales of the Reformation period.[2] Bourneville's book on Jeanne Fery illustrated the realm of multiple personalities connected with hysterical somnambulism.[3] Charcot himself defined and delimited the sphere of effectiveness of healing faith with maximum clinical precision in his own booklet.[4]

Bourneville also discussed religious stigmatization with reference to the contemporary case of Louise Lateau which, unlike Virchow, he did not dismiss as 'either fraud or miracle.'[5] Charcot had recognized various vasomotor disturbances as neurotic manifestations; what are now called *psychosomatic* effects. He was the first to describe in patients the rare condition *blue edema*— swelling with local cyanosis and hypothermia. He also diagnosed it retrospectively among Louise Coirin's symptoms.[6] In 1890, he showed his class an analogous condition produced in a subject by a hypnotic suggestion given four days previously. The symptom was in a mild form and was 'cured' on the spot, yielding within minutes to countersuggestion. But it was relevant to 'stigmatization' problems as encountered in Louise Lateau and others. A mottled blue swelling, the edema gave a bright red spot when touched.[7] Charcot had also noted in some patients the condition known as *autographic skin* which, if lightly impressed with a pencil, would soon appear intensely red.[8]

All these researches had the tendency of reducing the occult to the operation of natural forces, however imperfectly understood. But Charcot's vision was not limited, and he was prepared to admit in heaven and earth the existence of more things than were dreamt of in the natural philosophy of his time. No evidence is to hand of his own participation in psychical research. But during Charcot's last years, Axel Munthe was doing experiments at the Salpêtrière on telepathy and clairvoyance in the hypnotized.[9] As Munthe's association with the hospital was only peripheral, it can hardly be doubted that similar research was done there by other physicians with Charcot's knowledge and complaisance, even if he may have been reserved in assenting to conclusions.

In the 1880's, Janet communicated a report on the experiments in *psychologie supranormale* he had carried out on Léonie in a paper given Charcot's and Richet's Society for Physiological Psychology :

This little discourse, though very prudent and skeptical as to mental suggestion and hypnotism at a distance, nevertheless attracted the attention of the Society for Psychical Research in London who proposed to send one of their members to Le Havre to verify my work.[10]

In the event both F. W. H. Myers and his brother Dr A. T. Myers participated in the experiments, and the former certainly attended some of Charcot's lectures at the Salpêtrière.[11] Janet goes on to say :

My first entrance into the study of the disorders of the nervous system by examination of mysterious phenomena and the doubtful reality does not seem entirely regrettable. In the first place, these strange investigations have put me in contact with some

213

important people who had the same curiosity at the back of their minds, Charcot, Charles Richet, Frederick Myers, Sidgwick. They have informed me of their own enthusiasms and doubts. . . . This difficult and dangerous research work has taught me from the beginning the necessity of a certain disposition of mind indispensable for the study of pathological psychology. One must approach this research with a certain calmness devoid of systematic and predetermined admiration or denial. Charcot said to me later in speaking of the study of hysteria '*Nil admirari* is an indispensable attitude.'[12]

Clearly, Charcot would have thought appropriate to the study of the paranormal the same empirical undogmatic attitude he had brought to hysteria. He knew that one cannot legislate for Nature, and that the outcome of research cannot be known in advance. From Charcot's own triumph in reducing the facts of hysteria from chaos to comparative order, we can learn that in parapsychology we are not entitled to premature despair because its phenomena are capricious or under suspicion of fraud, or because its subject matter consists of dispersed and seemingly unrelated fragments. 'Hysteria has its laws,' Charcot asserted, in concert with Hippocrates who affirmed that epilepsy belonged to the natural order. With these exemplars it would be foolish to assume that laws of parapsychology are not there to be found in the fullness of time, if we take our cue from Charcot and are prepared to collect, analyze, and compare inchoate data until—looked at with a steady eye—they yield to reason.

In preceding pages we have found much to refute the gratuitous assumption that Charcot 'thought only in terms of brain and nerves.' Instead, he can be considered a proponent of 'psychophysical parallelism' as a pragmatic approach to the complexities of the 'mind-brain' problem. No theoretical exposition of his standpoint is found in his printed works other than the statement of 1867, that a correspondence and not an antagonism must exist between vital and physical properties. But, as we have seen, Charcot tended more and more to describe the facts of hysteria in mental terms while at the same time admitting the 'grey matter' of the cerebral cortex as the seat of psychical events. His parallelism of language was a pragmatic approach quite befitting one who, in his youth, had been impressed with the 'positive philosophy' of Comte. Positivism emphasizes the relativity of knowledge and the changing evolving nature of every scientific discipline. Consequently the 'positive' approach, when not pushed to unjustified extremes, is a kind of scientific pragmatism, consciously making do with working hypotheses and intellectual expedients whose validity is recognized as transient. When dealing with neurological disease, Charcot could speak in terms of ganglia and gyri. But he tended to speak in mental terms when referring to the etiology of neuroses. For him the gulf between these two descriptions was not to be regarded as destined to be absolute and impassable, but it was the best that could be done at the time, and little better can be done now. In respect of parallelism as a working hypothesis, Charcot can be considered a predecessor of his compatriots Flournoy and Claparède.[13]

The latter psychologist, Claparède, gave as the guiding principles in his own life—Liberalism, Pragmatism, and Protestantism. This triad applies also to Charcot if we enlarge Protestantism to mean freedom of thought and expression.[14] His pragmatism in natural philosophy had, as its counterpart, agnosticism in religion. He appreciated virtue in individuals irrespective of their religion or lack of it. His *patron* Rayer had failed to be admitted as a Professor of the *Agrégation*, being ineligible as the husband of a Protestant. Hence Charcot was no lover of the Catholic church in its social and political aspects, but religion did not detract from friendship except with those who menaced the Republic and the tolerance, social progress, and intellectual freedom it symbolized. Many of his friends were freethinkers of a more militant kind, among them Brouardel, a pioneer in public health and a founder-member of the *Société des Penseurs-Libres*, and Bourneville, who wished to place social services under secular control. Charcot's step-son-in-law, Waldeck-Rousseau, became after Charcot's death one of the strongest Prime Ministers France ever had, a firm upholder of the civil power, who disciplined the clerical party and the military after the Dreyfus affair. Had Charcot been alive, it is likely that he would have been a Dreyfusard, because no anti-Semitism can be detected in him, and the Dreyfusards became identified with defense of the Republic against clericalism, dictatorship, and monarchism. Claparède, visiting the Salpêtrière in 1898, found Charcot's successor Dejerine isolated as an anti-Dreyfusard, the rest of the staff and the interns being fervently for Dreyfus.[15]

Charcot was basically a happy man, possessed of a placidly optimistic outlook in his private life. Hence it would be misleading to say he took a somber view of life. But, as a student of incurable organic diseases he could not be Dr Pangloss and ignore the grim face of destiny. He could, when moved by tragedy, quote Shakespeare to the effect that humans are to the gods like flies to wanton boys. Yet he did not reject life as 'gloom all-way.' On the last day of his life, as recounted by Pasteur's son-in-law, Vallery-Radot, he referred to de Maupassant's work as that of a sick man. 'The world is better, there is more goodness.' When the conversation took a philosophical turn he said: 'For me there is a God, but far, far away, very vague.'

CHAPTER X

Citizen Charcot

FREUD SAID of Charcot that he had 'a perfectly honest human delight in his own great success.'[1] This argues for a certain natural modesty—a tendency to render thanks to Fortune rather than to accept it all as his due. According to Freud, Charcot used to speak freely about his early days and the road he had traversed.

Only ten years after Waterloo, Jean-Martin was born in a house, now demolished, attached to his father's shop whose window displayed sketches of the brightly colored, high-perched carriages fashionable at that time. This was at 1 Rue du Faubourg Poissonière, near the present Conservatoire de Musique and just north of the present Boulevard Poissonière—one of the chain of boulevards stretching from the Madeleine to the Place de la République. Charcot *père* had but recently worked his way up from being a wheelwright, and his means were limited. He therefore sent each of his four sons for one year to the Lycée Bonaparte, with the intention that whichever one obtained the best recommendation from the teachers should continue there. This proved easily to be Jean-Martin. His resolve to become a medical student seems to have proceeded indirectly from his love of animals. He would watch the treatments being given to the patients at a veterinary surgeon's premises that lay on his route to and from the Lycée.

Charcot's early medical career has already been described in outline. In retrospect the decisive event can be recognized as happening in 1853, when he was twenty-eight years old and Rayer's *Chef de Clinique* at *La Pitié*. Rayer, despite the academic misadventure resulting from his marriage, was then physician to Prince Jerome Napoleon, the son of the erstwhile Bonapartist King of Westphalia, and was developing influence through his acquaintance with Louis Napoleon who had become Emperor in 1852 as a result of the coup d'état in the preceding autumn, ratified by popular referendum. It was to Rayer's good offices that Charcot partly owed his appointment as *Médecin* and *Chéf e Clinique* at the Salpêtrière in 1856, his professorship of the *Agrégation*, and finally after Rayer had been made dean of the Faculty, his longed for appointment as *Médecin de l'Hospice de la Salpêtrière*. But it was also Rayer who started Charcot off in private practice. Charcot at that time was adorned with a moustache. 'You will never have a patient,' said Rayer, 'until you dispense with it.'[2] Charcot declared he would cut it off as soon as Rayer found him a patient. A few days later Rayer wrote to say the moustache could go because Charcot now had a patient. This was Fould, a banker himself and the brother of a banker who was Napoleon's Minister of Finance. Minister Fould was a shrewd financier who prospered (like the Rothschilds) by not being too greedy and therefore 'sold too early.' One of Napoleon's other ministers who had ruined himself by rash buying after the coup d'état complained to the Emperor that Fould had instead reckoned on a panic and had gained by selling. Of Fould it is said that he maintained an opinion, considered eccentric in the rather dizzy speculative circles of Second Empire Paris, that the only source of real wealth was hard work.

Charcot's Fould had been advised by Rayer to take a trip to Italy for the sake of his health, accompanied by Charcot as physician. They penetrated as far as Naples, visiting all the celebrated centers of art and architecture en route. Charcot returned enriched by several folios of his own sketches, a handsome fee from Fould, and the permanent friendship of the family who remained his patients. He set up a small consulting room in the Rue Laffitte, which extends from Nôtre Dame de Lorette (in the district of cheap appartments, giving its name to the 'lorettes'—ladies of easy virtue) southward to the Crédit Lyonnais and the Opéra Comique. This modest beginning led eventually to the most celebrated private practice in Europe.

Those were exciting days in Paris. The life of the boulevardiers; journalists, actors, the beau monde, the dandies, and the jeunesse dorée had been long established, and the gaiety of life in the capital had been accepted with proverbial authority. Offenbach arrived in 1833, but the can-can, a wild dance imported from Algeria, had become fashionable the year before. Twenty years later the gaiety was to continue, but within an enlarged setting of change and progress in which the ordinary citizen might find a sense of drama and optimism. The new Emperor, faced with a variety of insoluble paradoxes in the political and economic life of the country, had to do something for the workers, the peasants, and the bourgeoisie, all of whom agreed only in regarding their interests as mutually opposing. As a result, Napoleon had to set in motion an endless cycle of adjustments. Steps to benefit industrial workers were resented by the bourgeoisie, who had to be placated in their turn. Thus the Emperor, though totally innocent of any radical intentions, became the instrument of widespread social change. Funds for better workers' housing and legislation for friendly societies, savings banks, workmen's compensation, legal and medical assistance for the poor were balanced by railway concessions, encouragement of shipping, and cheap credit, and the *paysans* benefited from drainage and afforestation schemes, agricultural loans and insurance, and the organization of 'chambers of agriculture.'

The rebuilding of Paris was one of Napoleon's favorite projects not, as is sometimes said, so that revolts could be conveniently suppressed with artillery, but for the worthy aims of hygiene, traffic flow, and the combating of unemployment as well as to be a personal monument and a good advertisement. In 1853, the year that Charcot joined Rayer, Napoleon appointed Baron Haussmann, a ruthless and efficient autocrat, to be Prefect of the Seine. Assisted by the engineer Alphand, Haussmann's aim was that the city be laid out like one immense park, with gardens and landscaped woodlands linked by splendid and leafy boulevards radiating from monuments and *rondes*. The final result was 'the first modern city since the Rome of the Caesars.'[3] Haussmann's improvements brought the whole world to the capital, which seemed natural enough to the Parisians, for 'in the minds of the boulevardiers, all travel was in a subjective direction, towards Paris.'⁴ In the meantime there were immense piles of debris, innumerable buildings under construction, and a great influx of population. The vast work was achieved, but the finances of the capital were brought to bankruptcy. More seriously the destruction of slums, done impartially in all quarters of the city, though an excellent thing in itself, destroyed the propinquity in which all classes—artisans and aristocrats—had dwelled side by side in the old Faubourgs. High rents drove the working people from the center of the city, where the bourgeoisie and the boulevardiers, augmented by an inflow of plutocratic cosmopolitans, lived the ever gayer and more dream-like existence satirized by Offenbach in *La Vie Parisienne*.

But the life of undiluted pleasure was mainly confined to the boulevards of the Right Bank. 'Society' as such seems to have attracted Charcot little even in his later days of eminence and prosperity. His preference inclined to the more solid and placid. Through his artistic interests he fell in with a well-to-do art collector, the owner of a tailoring business, M. Laurent Richard. Charcot frequently dined at Richard's comfortable villa in the Avenue de Madrid at Neuilly. Here Charcot met Richard's young widowed daughter Mme Augustine Victoire Durvis, described as a good-looking girl with blue eyes and a figure slightly plumper than was considered fashionable at the time. Augustine had a small daughter, Marie Durvis, aged seven and very pretty. M. Richard was a connoisseur of men as well as of paintings and very fond of Charcot. He was more than content to approve Charcot's marriage to Augustine, which he regarded as a perfectly equitable match. Indeed, though Charcot's origins were modest and his wealth as yet meager, it would have been foolish to have regarded him as a fortune hunter. As a *Médecin* of the Paris hospitals with a private practice well launched, Charcot had in effect a licence to coin money, had he wished to exploit it. In the event the fortune he left to his only son Jean amounted to 400,000 francs, a goodly sum but by no means excessive for one of the world's most famous physicians.

Charcot married a little prior to 1862, being still only a *Chef de Clinique* at the Salpêtrière. The moustache had come and gone. He was only in his thirties and a reliable idea of his appearance, which was undeniably handsome in an unpretentious and restrained kind of way, can be derived from the only known likeness of him in his earlier years. This is one of the medallions adorning the physicians' lounge at La Charité and represents Charcot at the age of twenty-three. The face is moderately elongated and 'strong,' though reposed, and with a hint of slightly ironic humor. The forehead is high and square, the jaw and cheekbones are powerful. The lack of portraits of Charcot in his mature years is a little odd and presumably an effect of chance. It is less surprising for his early life, when photography was a rare art. Even in 1859, when Charcot was thirty-four, photography was so novel that Louis Napoleon, departing at the head of his troops for the Italian campaign, and noticing a photographer, halted the whole cavalcade and posed while it waited.[5]

Laurent Richard was generous to the newly wedded couple who acquired an apartment in the Avenue du Coq off the Rue St Lazare, near to the Opéra and the new Boulevard Hauss-mann. Augustine Victoire is said to have been a woman of firm mind, but tactful in handling her single-minded husband to whose interests she was dedicated. She was an incomplete feminist. Their first child Jeanne, born in 1865, was reared on goat's milk, but when their second and last infant, Jean, arrived, Madame declared that goat's milk was good enough only for a girl.[6] This was in 1867, when they rented a villa at Neuilly, now a suburb of Paris but then a country place. On the walls of the villa they inscribed quotations from their favorite authors and a proverb: '*A chacun oysel son nid si semble bel.*' ('To every bird its nest seems beautiful'). At 29 Rue St James they were near to Laurent Richard and almost in sight of the black swans on the Mare de St James in the Bois de Boulogne, formerly a wilderness but by then landscaped into a park.

The year 1867—this brings us to where we came in, to meet Charcot in the little ward kitchen, adapted as a lecture room. It was a significant year not only in the history of medicine, but in the history of France. It was the year of the World Exhibition, represented by the huge building on the Champ de Mars crowded with every kind of machinery and indicative of the industrial development and growth of trade the Emperor had very properly encouraged. Idealists dreamed of universal peace brought about as a result of social progress and the spread of liberty and enlightenment. Victor Hugo predicted that the next century would see the birth of a great and peaceful nation whose capital would be Paris and whose name would be Europe. Hopes were good for freedom in France. Though the Empire might continue, the dictatorship could only be temporary. The structure of politics had changed since 1848. Solid middle-class and even republican working-class opinion was tiring of the doctrinaire purism of the older generation of revolutionaries and socialists; it looked to parliamentary democracy with constitutional government by an Emperor with reduced authority—a French 'Queen Victoria'; it supported the Republican Opposition elected to the Chamber of Deputies in 1863. This new generation had Charcot's friend Gambetta as its most emphatic leader. The Opposition opposed Napoleon's wasteful Mexican adventure. It won concessions for the workers and the rights of trade union organization. On his part, the Emperor became increasingly more liberal. Correspondingly, the haute bourgeoisie, as opposed to the reformist bourgeoisie, lived an even more fin du siècle existence in an atmosphere reminiscent of a century before—*après nous le déluge*—as expressed in Offenbach's *La Belle Hélène*.

It was said by Zilboorg that to Charcot, 'history was like the weather' and hardly noticed.[7] But this is rather less than the full truth. At the end of his 1867 lectures, Charcot drew approving attention to the recent development of German science. 'We have realized that a great scientific power has just arisen next to us.' He next administered a rebuke to some German savants. 'Our neighbours, drunk with their success, appear to have persuaded themselves that the whole domain of science belongs henceforth to them.' This can be understood and condoned, says Charcot, but,

> it is not without regret that we have seen not long ago an eminent man confuse the rights, which were bestowed upon him by virtue of his high position as a scientist, with the political mandate given by the electors of Berlin, and abuse the word 'Science' just in order to propagandize German intellectuals towards a narrow patriotism.

Charcot then, 'against the unliberal and exclusive ideas of this Prussian scientist,' opposed the words of 'a great English physician' [Robert James Graves] to the effect that 'reason had the entire world for its domain.'[9] (Robert James Graves was grandfather of the distinguished poet Robert von Ranke Graves, whose other grandfather was Heinrich von Ranke, a radical who had to leave Prussia temporarily in 1848 for demonstrating against the government).

The curious fact was that the offender castigated so magisterially by Charcot happened to be, in German terms, someone very much like Charcot himself. It was Virchow, the brilliant pathologist and man of many interests, who was also a liberal and an opponent of the political and cultural influence of the Catholics. Like Bourneville, whose interest in public health eventually put him on the Paris Municipal Council, Virchow entered politics and opposed Bismarck's policy of unifying Germany through a series of wars. Even so, his relatively minor indiscretion illustrates the nationalistic tendency of the German liberals in the nineteenth century. Charcot's own patriotism was of an innocent kind. Freud remarks that Charcot disliked the German reaction to his announcement of the occurrence of hysteria in men, which was to the effect that it was confined to Frenchmen. He was, therefore, delighted when a case described as 'reflex epilepsy' in a Prussian grenadier could be diagnosed by him at a distance as one of hysteria.[10]

Charcot's strictures on Virchow, though possibly more strict than was warranted, echoed accurately enough the forebodings felt by intelligent Parisians in that time of hope and glory. Only the year before Bismarck, in whom there was more than a touch of the hysterical somnambulist, had learned in a dream that a fratricidal war between Germany and Austria was the divinely appointed solution to his political problems. The revelation was put briskly into effect by using the new railroads to concentrate troops. The most brilliant success of the year of the Exhibition was Offenbach's *Grand Duchess of Gerolstein*, a multisided satire lampooning at one and the same time both German and French militarism in the figure of 'General Boum,' and Bismarck's labryinthine policy in the figure of 'Baron Puck.' The performances were attended by everyone who was anyone in the grand monde or the demi-monde. Louis Napoleon smiled wryly at the Picrocholean military plans of General Boum. The Prince of Wales took the first steps toward the Entente Cordiale by visiting the leading lady, Hortense Schneider, in her dressing room. But the visitor who most appreciated the operetta was Bismarck himself—Baron Puck in person.

Bismarck returned three years later. The Emperor was a prisoner. At Versailles the King of Prussia was declared German Emperor. Thiers and Gambetta proclaimed the Third Republic. Paris was surrounded and enduring its first siege. Gambetta escaped by balloon to raise new armies. Bismarck settled at Versailles to keep everything under control, especially the Kaiser! To get a quick result, he insisted on the bombardment of the city. Charcot wrote to his exiled family that the shells came at the rate of two shots a minute and that a monument should be erected to the shame of Germany. The letters had to be written in minute handwriting on very thin paper and conveyed by balloon, but they were peppered with jokes to keep Madame Charcot's spirits up. The family, with Laurent Richard, went to Dieppe until, on the arrival there of 10,000 German occupying troops, they were persuaded by their friends, the Italian-born Casellas family, to join them at Upper Phillimore Gardens, Kensington, London. Charcot remained in Paris. All teaching and research were suspended. The Salpêtrière, besides catering for its normal inmates, was pressed into service as a hospital for casualties and the victims of the curent smallpox and typhoid epidemics. At one period, for lack of other transport, Charcot had to travel to the hospital by boat. His armband as a casualty officer was worn again by Jeanne when in ambulance service in the 1914 war.

The winter of 1870 was very severe. Gambetta's armies in the country were winning successes, and the Germans might have had to break off the siege had not the commanders in Paris surrendered on January 28, 1871. On March 18 the Commune took over the city and the German army, still encamped on the heights around, watched its second siege, conducted this time by a French army reconstituted by Thiers. Gambetta had left the government, which desired a peace treaty with Germany while he wished to continue the struggle. The witticism that Paris is so revolutionary a city that the very cobblestones rise from the ground refers to the 'barricades' of 1848 and 1870. Louis Gallet, the administrator of the Salpêtrière in 1871, wrote :

Dr Charcot arrived every morning for work. He came in an open carriage, looking very calm, and very cold as usual, with his thin, cleanly shaven face, long black hair and Napoleonic profile. He described how he was stopped by soldiers of the Commune while they . . . were building a barricade across the street and how he was able to get by them in spite of the protests of those who wished to force him to get out of his carriage and lift some paving stones for the barricade, which was the traditional toll exacted in times of insurrection.[11]

In May the army fought its way into the city. Numerous atrocities were alleged of the *Communards*, some of which had in fact been committed by psychopaths among them. However vengeance was exacted a hundredfold in the greatest massacre in French history. The cemetery of Père Lachaise was the scene of events far more terrible than had ever troubled Saint Médard.

Charcot maintained the neutrality of a *Médecin* throughout it all, giving aid where it was needed. The Commune had no program and could not have seemed to offer any realistic government to France, and Charcot did not wish it to triumph. On the other hand, he had no desire for a return to monarchy—Bourbon, Orléanist, or Bonapartist—and it is likely that he viewed the government of Thiers, an ancient Orléanist, with 'modified rapture.' Still, normal life and work had to be resumed. By 1872, when Charcot became Professor of Pathological Anatomy, research and teaching were in full swing at the Salpêtrière. Madame Charcot and the three children returned to Paris in 1871, relieved not to find their house and apartment looted. A Welsh nursemaid had replaced her German predecessor, who had irritated Madame by exulting in the military successes of her compatriots. As for Charcot, he refused henceforth to attend medical congresses in Germany. Ireland, though Catholic, was a different matter. Although he detested religious intolerance, he himself was tolerant of all religions. In 1872,

Charcot was invited to Ireland as a member of a delegation of distinguished Frenchmen. Since he dressed in black like all Victorian physicians and all professional Frenchmen and had a dignified mien, the Irish addressed him as 'Your Reverence.' But religious questions were submerged in shared republican sentiment. The Dubliners hung out the 'green' and the Tricolor and whistled the 'Marseillaise' and 'Erin-go-Brach.'

Madame Charcot, however, had seen enough of the world and did not wish to go on her travels again. With her the urge to hygiene assumed phobic proportions; when she traveled she had to take her bedding, her washbasin, and extensive baggage. Realizing that she was a poor companion away from home she encouraged Jean-Martin to travel on his own.

Charcot's marriage was undoubtedly a perfectly happy one. He was not flirtatious. Indeed, he was so little of a philanderer that Axel Munthe almost makes it into a fault. 'Sharing the fate of all nerve specialists he was surrounded by a body-guard of neurotic ladies, hero-worshipers at all costs. Luckily for him he was absolutely indifferent to women.'[12] As a matter of fact it is difficult to see (if Munthe is correct) where Charcot would meet all these women, other than as private patients in his consulting room. Charcot did not go into society as such. Thursday evenings were devoted to music. On Tuesday evenings there was an 'At Home,' attended mainly by Charcot's medical colleagues, family friends, and various artistic acquaintances. It is very likely that Charcot's usual reserve and shyness came into play with ladies as it did with anyone he did not know well. It is probable also that, like many another savant, he had been a serious and dedicated youth, unpracticed as a ladies' man, and possibly needed a young lady such as Augustine Victoire, already thawed by marriage to 'bring him out'. But there is ample testimony that in relaxed surroundings with those he knew, whether at work or at home, he was a genial and fluent talker possessed of warmth and wit. Freud testifies concerning his relationship with his Salpêtrians :

> Some members of this circle of young men whom he had gathered about him and made his partners in his work had attained to consciousness of their own individuality, . . . and one

or other of them would now and then advance an opinion that seemed to the master clever rather than correct; this he would attack sarcastically enough in conversation and in his lectures without, however, in any way injuring his affectionate relation with the pupil.

. . . an academic teacher of intellectual importance is not also automatically gifted with that close personal influence on his students which expresses itself in the formation of a numerous and important 'school.' If Charcot was more favoured in this respect we must attribute it to his personal qualities as a man, to the magic of his aspect and his voice, to the gracious frankness of his manner after the first strangeness of a new relation had worn off, to the readiness with which he placed everything at the disposal of his pupils, and to his life-long loyalty to them. The hours he spent in his wards were hours of fellowship and interchange of ideas with his whole medical staff. He never shut himself off from them; the youngest assistant had an opportunity of seeing him at work and might interrupt him, and the same privilege was granted to the foreigners who were never absent from his rounds in later years. Finally, his pupils and assistants were regarded as part of his family in welcoming the guests on the evenings when Madame Charcot . . . received a distinguished company in her hospitable house.[13]

By way of a lighthearted tribute to the little doctor's attractiveness, we have the lines addressed to him impromptu by Garnier, the architect of the Paris Opera House and a frequent visitor to the Charcot ménage, warning the ladies that Charcot might entrance them with hypnotic passes, but 'I must say, he could easily keep them awake.'[14] Charcot felt a sort of fatherly responsibility for his pupils, who called him *Patron* as did all the Charcot family. Madame Charcot was *la patronne*, helping the interns in their trials and tribulations. According to Georges Guinon, 'When we wished to get something from the boss [*patron*] and were doubtful of his acquiescence, we always begged Madame Charcot to make our request for us. And it would always succeed if we did not ask for the impossible.' Occasionally, Charcot would take a party of interns to the Folies Bergères to cheer them up. This was not so bad as it sounds, for 'Les Girls' were not brought to the Folies till 1894, by which time Charcot was dead.

When the fighting was over in 1871, the Charcot family settled in a spacious apartment in the Hôtel de Chimay, an elegant seventeenth-century building, now the *École des Beaux Arts*. Situated on the Quai Malaquais, it looked across the Seine to the Louvre. Charcot was often to be seen strolling with his hands behind him browsing at the bookstalls along the Quai. As playmates Jean and Jeanne Charcot had the children of Edouard Pailleron, the writer, who also occupied an apartment in the Hôtel de Chimay. In the summer months they still went to their villa at Neuilly. The first voyage of Jean Charcot, the great explorer, was in a soap-box, christened the 'Pourquoi Pas?' on the Mare St James. Attacked by the black swans and letting in water, the vessel foundered. When young Jean was nine, his father, looking for a nonsectarian school, found one in the École Alsacienne near the Observatory, and Jean traveled there daily from Neuilly and back on an aged *diligence*.

Meanwhile Charcot attended the Salpêtrière every morning (except Good Friday, it is said) with a regularity that became proverbial. At the stroke of nine he would arrive in his landau, driven by the same coachman Robert for twenty-five years. To avoid waste of time he would be reading and might need a tap on the window to tell him he had arrived. He would pat the horses' noses and give them a piece of bread brought for the purpose. He would then go in to meet his assembled interns, the *Chefs de Clinique*, and the Chief Nurse of the Pariset Division, Mlle Botard, who had entered the nursing service in 1835, at a wage of eight francs a month, when the working day was sixteen hours long. In the afternoon Charcot would receive patients at his private consulting rooms. His anteroom was always thronged with Parisians and with patients 'from Samarcand and from the Antilles' as Freud puts it, who also says:

> This throng was assuredly not attracted merely by the famous scientist, but as much or more by the great physician, and by the sympathetic nature of the man, who always knew how to give counsel, and could surmise and guess in those cases where the present status of science did not permit him to know.[15]

The consultation fee was the same for all patients who could pay it—40 francs. But all who knew Charcot well, particularly Pierre Marie and Georges Guinon who assisted at the consulting room, say that he never refused free consultations to those of limited means, or made them delay their turn for the benefit of a celebrity. One day a princess was annoyed at having to wait with other patients. Charcot merely pitied the foreigner who did not know that the Bastille had fallen.

In 1884, when he had arrived at the summit of his profession, Charcot acquired a beautiful house at 217 Boulevard Saint-Germain, built in 1704 as 'l'Hôtel Varengeville.' Situated in the intersection of the Boulevard and the Rue Saint-Dominique, it stood in a district that still comprised a wide variety of residents. Intellectuals and writers such as Charcot's friend Alphonse Daudet, who lived opposite to him, rubbed shoulders with aristo-crats and bourgeoisie, and even blacksmiths. The sound of a forge could be heard at both Daudet's and Charcot's houses. They made a pact that the one who lived the longer should remember the other whenever he heard the familiar sound. Daudet survived Charcot by five years and would say 'Alas, Charcot' when he heard the clang of the hammers. The mansion was furnished luxuriously to Charcot's visual taste, which inclined to the medieval : tapestries, stained-glass windows, wrought-iron chandeliers, wood paneling and dark wooden columns, and furniture of sculptured woodwork. Charcot's study was an imposing but well-proportioned room. In later years the Hôtel Varengeville became the premises of the Bank of Algeria, but the books and furnishings were set up at the Salpêtrière as the Charcot Library. The books were housed in large bookcases and in a gallery reached by two winding staircases, the design being based on the Library of the Medici at Florence. The stained-glass windows gave a somewhat 'dim religious light.' The study was also Charcot's consulting room where, sitting behind a large desk, he received patients who were liable to be some-what awed by the surroundings and the inscrutable mask of the Professor.

Charcot would never dine out; he went only to concerts or to the opera. Every Tuesday, however, guests were invited to dinner which was followed by an 'At Home' to which were invited Salpêtrians, other scientists such as Pasteur, and numerous artists and writers as well as philosophers and psychologists such as Ribot, Jules Janet, and Charles Richet. Entertainments were provided for children of all ages—games, charades, recitations. Among the political figures seen at the Charcots' was Dom Pedro, the Emperor of Brazil who would often play billiards with the Professor. A liberal and a man of the highest character, he had republican sympathies. Among more obvious 'Jacobins' were Gambetta, and Naquet, something of an agitator, responsible for introducing legal divorce into France : he was the patient for whose rheumatism Charcot prescribed a bag of warm oats. Waldeck-Rousseau is said to have been rather bored by the animated talk on art, literature, and philosophy which often went on at these soirées. Described as one of Gambetta's young 'marshals' and destined to be Premier, Waldeck-Rousseau was the second husband of Marie Durvis, Charcot's stepdaughter. Marie first married Dr Liouville, one of Charcot's interns and later a professor, who died young leaving a son, another medical, Jacques Liouville. Marie was always on the closest terms of affection with her half-siblings and was devoted to Jean Charcot. With very distinguished good looks, she is described as being always the 'Prime Ministress.'

The bond between Charcot and Louis Pasteur was close. In 1887, Pasteur's anti-rabic vaccine was under severe attack in the Academy of Medicine. Pasteur himself was ill and away in Italy. Professor Peter claimed that the vaccine, so far from curing rabies, caused it. Charcot went down to Pasteur's laboratory, carefully questioned Pasteur's assistants, examined the experimental records, and went away silently. At the Academy of Medicine, he quoted the words of Vulpian (who had died a few months previously) that Pasteur's experimental genius had resulted in one of the most beautiful discoveries ever made— whether considered from a scientific or a humanitarian viewpoint.

Charcot loved to travel. 'Movement does me a great deal of good. It is definitely the treatment for me. It is a great thing to learn and to enjoy oneself at the same time.' He visited all Europe, always preparing himself in advance by studying the history, archeology, and way of life of the country he intended to visit. He visited all the great museums and also the markets and populous districts 'in order better to understand the customs of the inhabitants.' In 1883, with Jean and Jeanne, who from then on always accompanied him, he penetrated the wild recesses of Wales, where much of the journey had to be accomplished by stagecoach. On occasion the coachman was drunk and they careened from side to side in the descent of a wild mountain pass. Once they stayed in Moscow with the Poliakoff family who had built the railway from Moscow to Saint Petersburg. As democrats the Charcots were horrified by the ways of the *ancien régime* which required that servants sleep all night on the floors of the corridors in case they were required. Charcot's own house was one of the first in Paris to supply a bathroom for the servants. Charcot had been summoned to Russia in 1873 to give the Tsar a medical opinion. Once Gambetta, wishing to explore the possibility of an entente with Russia, asked Charcot to invite the Grand Duke Nicholas to the house at Neuilly. After an informal conversation lasting two hours, Gambetta and the Duke rejoined the company for dinner. Embarrassment and then amusement resulted from the discovery that the pet monkey Rosalie had taken bites out of the dessert apples.

The children grew up. Marie was married. Jeanne, a very good-looking girl with keen blue eyes and an independent nature, having been brought up rather as a boy among boys with Jean and his friends, was known as Mlle Pallas. Each child had a separate suite in one of the wings of the great house. The family shared a large studio where Madame Charcot and Jeanne worked in clay, leather, glass and metal. Jeanne won a medal for a statuette in the Exhibition of 1900. The Professor drew, carved wood, or painted pottery which the ladies themselves baked and glazed. Jean characteristically drew ships. For summer holidays they often went to Ouistreham where Jean could 'mess about in boats,' fraternize with the fishermen, and learn to handle a ship. Another family hobby was cycling. Even Madame Charcot would participate, though heavily veiled to avoid recognition, when on Sundays they cycled to Barbizon. Charcot hazarded himself on a tricycle.

Jean yearned passionately to join the navy and go to sea. His father is sometimes regarded as harsh and stern for insisting that his son study medicine. But Marthe Oulié, Jean's god-daughter who knew him very well, says that his father's real reason was that he could not bear the idea of Jean leaving home on long voyages. In the event, Charcot told Jean that he must get his medical qualification, after which he could do as he liked. He may have felt that Jean was capable of mastering an intellectual discipline and would ultimately profit by the effort. In a letter he wrote : 'You must get used to finding pleasure in work. It is a great joy to learn and understand . . . *to excel in something*.' Jean justified his father's belief in his capacities. He applied himself, became an extern at the Saint-Antoine, then an intern at the Salpêtrière, where Janet refers to him as having designed a device for measuring muscular tremor.[16] In 1895 he became Doctor of Medicine, his thesis being on 'Progressive Muscular Atrophy.' Under Charcot's successor, Raymond, he became *Chéf de Clinique*. Later he worked for a while at the Pasteur Institute.

In his student and intern days, Jean was gay. Sometimes he and his companions were arrested by the police for minor dis-orderliness. On one occasion the charge list read like the Pantheon—Berthelot, Charcot, Daudet. A practical joker, legal proceedings were once commenced against Jean for violating the law that *animaux féroces* must not be transported in cabs. The animal was Sigurd, the family St Bernard, disguised as a lion. Once he drove up to the very fashionable restaurant Château de Madrid in the gardener's cart drawn by Saladin, the donkey. One afternoon he astonished a crowd in the Bois de Boulogne by throwing into the water an elegant young lady who was with him in a boat on the Mare Saint James. When the police recovered the corpse it was found to be a scarecrow in Jeanne's clothes. One of his fellow students, Bouchacourt, good-natured but credulous, was invited on numerous occasions to meet His Imperial Highness the Grand Duke Boris, who was eventually revealed to be Cavelier, the son of a prosperous Paris grocer. Jean was a close friend of Léon Daudet's until the latter, having failed his medical finals, declared that Jean only passed because he was Charcot's son. Thereupon Jean terminated the friendship.

It is to Léon Daudet, however, that we owe a description of père Charcot relaxed with his friends on Tuesday evenings :

232

One could write a captivating story just by recording the conversations. . . . He was like Goethe, Montaigne, or Alphonse Daudet, like those men who radiate interest in everything. *Nihil humanum a me alienum puto* was his motto. . . . He hated banalities and the commonplace. He would excerpt from his vast readings items seeming to concern the destiny of man. . . .

It was a joy to listen to Charcot on these Tuesday evenings . . . while he was chatting about different things with my father (Alphonse Daudet), Phillipe Burty, and Arène, or concentrating his thoughts on one or another of the classical authors, and giving in a few words a striking description that also had depth and was unforgettable. How many times, . . . did I hear Alphonse Daudet, who carefully weighed his eulogies, repeat: 'Charcot is a genius.'[17]

Charcot continued his work unremittingly into his seventh decade, spending the forenoon at the hospital, the afternoon in his consulting room, and frequently sitting in his study writing late into the night. A good trencherman, he smoked cigars and a pipe. The bill for this regimen was first presented on New Year's Eve, 1890. After supper at which the children and some friends including Pasteur were present, Charcot suffered his first attack of angina. Professor Potain, Charcot's contemporary and his unique coequal as a clinician, was summoned. Two and a half years was the prognosis he gave privately to Léon Daudet. It was fulfilled with remarkable accuracy. In August 1893, at Madame Charcot's persuasion, Charcot went to Vézelay in Burgundy, accompanied by his pupils Debove, Straus, and Vallery-Radot. Visiting the famous Basilica, he pointed out, with some emotion, the dark chamber entered by a hole in the wall out of view of the altar, where the possessed were relegated in earlier days. He remarked of the tower that it was 'violent and brutal, like a citadel or prison. The walls seem to cry out, "Ill will to him who does not have faith".'[18] Two nights later he died suddenly at the auberge where they were staying.

Charcot's coffin was brought to the Salpêtrière where it lay in state preparatory to the funeral service which, in accordance with Charcot's wishes, was held in the hospital and took place without speeches. Pupils and patients raised a fund, half of which was contributed by foreign physicians, for a bronze statue of Charcot in academic robes. Executed by Charcot's friend, the sculptor Falguière, it stood at the hospital entrance along with that of Pinel.

The fame of the Charcot family reached its peak in 1925, when the Faculty of Medicine celebrated the centenary of his birth, with numerous *éloges* attended by delegates from all over the world. Jeanne and her husband Arthur Hendry (a Scottish relative of the Harmsworth family) received the Cross of the Legion of Honor for their war services. Tributes were also paid to the greatness of Jean Charcot, now a national hero in respect of his voyages of scientific exploration. Two years later he became a Commander of the Legion of Honor and a member of the Academy of Sciences. In 1936, on the eve of retirement from the sea, he was drowned with almost all his companions near Reyjavik when a gale sank the 'Pourquoi Pas?'—the successor to his first craft sunk in the Mare Saint James. The funeral ceremony was held in Nôtre Dame.

As for Professor Charcot, he died his second death in 1942 when the Germans took his statue for scrap metal. But along with the names of Mazarin, Vincent de Paul, and Pinel there remains inscribed over the gates of the Salpêtrière still the name of CHARCOT.

REFERENCES

Chapter I

[1] JEAN-MARTIN CHARCOT, *Lectures on Senile and Chronic Diseases* (London: New Sydenham Society, 1881), pp. 1-29.
[2] ROBERT GRAVES, *The Greek Myths* (London: Penguin Books, 1961), I, p. 115.
[3] *Ibid.*, I, p. 175.
[4] ERWIN ROHDE, *Psyche* (London: Kegan Paul, 1925).
[5] F. L. MARCUSE, *Hypnosis, Fact and Fiction* (London: Penguin Books, 1959).
[6] GREGORY ZILBOORG and G. W. HENRY, *A History of Medical Psychology* (New York: Norton, 1941), p. 559.
[7] BENJAMIN FARRINGTON, *Greek Science* (London: Penguin Books, 1961), p. 67.
E. T. WITHINGTON, 'The Asclepiadae and the Priests of Asclepius' in Charles Singer, ed., *Studies in the History and Methods of Science*, II (1921), pp. 192-205.
[8] W. H. S. JONES, trans., *Hippocrates* (London: Heinemann, Loeb Classical Library, n.d.).
[9] FARRINGTON, *op. cit.*, p. 151.
[10] WALTER A. JAYNE, *The Gods of Ancient Civilizations* (New Haven: Yale University Press, 1925).
[11] CHARCOT, *op. cit.*, p. 17.
[12] *Loc. cit.*
[13] *Loc. cit.*
[14] ZILBOORG and HENRY, *op. cit.*, p. 251.
[15] CHARCOT, *op. cit.*, p. 17.
[16] *Ibid.*, p. 18.
[17] ZILBOORG and HENRY, *op. cit.*, p. 116.
[18] *Ibid.*, pp. 562-63.
[19] ALDOUS HUXLEY, *The Devils of Loudun* (London: Chatto and Windus, 1952), p. 341.
[20] CHARLES M. CAMPBELL, *Destiny and Disease in Mental Disorders* (London: Chapman & Hall, 1935), p. 17.
[21] *Loc. cit.*
[22] GEORGES GUILLAIN, *J.-M. Charcot. His Life—His Work* (London: Pitman Medical Publishing Company, 1959), p. 42.
ZILBOORG and HENRY, *op. cit.*, pp. 317-18.
[23] *Ibid.*, pp. 322-23.

Chapter II

[1] GEORGES GUILLAIN, *J.-M. Charcot. His Life—His Work* (London: Pitman Medical Publishing Company, 1959), p. 83.
[2] *Loc. cit.*
[3] *Ibid.*, p. 22.
[4] SIGMUND FREUD, 'Charcot', *Collected Papers* (London: Hogarth Press, 1948), I, p. 10.
[5] GUILLAIN, *op. cit.*, p. 7.
[6] *Ibid.*, p. 52.
[7] J.-M. CHARCOT, *Clinical Lectures on the Diseases of the Nervous System* (London: New Sydenham Society, 1889), III, p. 23.
[8] AXEL MUNTHE, *The Story of San Michele* (London: Murray, 1936), p. 205.
[9] *Ibid.*, p. 16.
[10] FREUD, *op. cit.*, pp. 10-11.
[11] *Loc. cit.*
[12] GUILLAIN, *op. cit.*, p. 89.
[13] *Ibid.*, p. 112.
[14] *Ibid.*, p. 120.
[15] *Loc. cit.*
[16] MUNTHE, *op. cit.*, p. 206.
[17] FREUD, *op. cit.*, p. 17.
[18] MUNTHE, *op. cit.*, p. 205.
[19] GUILLAIN, *op. cit.*, p. 117.
[20] *Ibid.*, p. 1,10.
[21] MUNTHE, *op. cit.*, p. 205.
[22] J.-M. CHARCOT and PIERRE MARIE, 'Hysteria' in D. Hack Tuke, ed., *Dictionary of Psychological Medicine* (London: Churchill, 1892), I, p. 629.
[23] GUILLAIN, *op. cit.*, p. 99.
[24] *Loc. cit.*
[25] FREUD, *op. cit.*, p. 14.
[26] *Ibid.*, p. 15.
[27] *Ibid.*, p. 16.
[28] GUILLAIN, *op. cit.*, p. 25.
[29] GUILLAIN, *op. cit.*, p. 166.
[30] CHARCOT, *Lectures on Senile and Chronic Diseases* (London: New Sydenham Society, 1881), p. 4.

Chapter III

[1] CHARCOT, *Clinical Lectures on the Diseases of the Nervous System* (London: New Sydenham Society, 1889), III, p. 12.
[2] AXEL MUNTHE, *The Story of San Michele* (London: Murray, 1936), p. 23.
[3] SIGMUND FREUD, *An Autobiographical Study* (London: Hogarth Press, 1935), pp. 19-20.
[4] GREGORY ZILBOORG and G. W. HENRY, *A History of Medical Psychology* (New York: Norton, 1941), p. 441.
[5] GEORGES GUILLAIN, *J.-M. Charcot. His Life—His Work* (London: Pitman Medical Publishing Company, 1959), p. 135.

[6] *Ibid.*, p. 144.
[7] ZILBOORG and HENRY, *op. cit.*, p. 260.
[8] PIERRE JANET, *The Major Symptoms of Hysteria* (New York: Macmillan, 1907), pp. 13-14.
[9] CHARCOT, *op. cit.*, p. 13.
[10] ZILBOORG and HENRY, *op. cit.*, pp. 362-364.
[11] FREUD, *op. cit.*, p. 23.
[12] SIGMUND FREUD, 'On the History of the Psycho-Analytical Movement,' *Collected Papers*, (London: Hogarth Press, 1948), I, pp. 287-359.
[13] J.-M. CHARCOT and PIERRE MARIE, 'Hysteria' in D. Hack Tuke, ed., *Dictionary of Psychological Medicine* (London: Churchill, 1892), I. p. 630.
[14] JANET, *op. cit.*, p. 21.
[15] *Loc. cit.*
[16] CHARCOT and MARIE, *op. cit.*, p. 633.
[17] JANET, *op. cit.*, p. 178.
[18] CHARCOT and MARIE, *op. cit.*, p. 635.
[19] ARTURO CASTIGLIONI, *A History of Medicine* (New York: Knopf, 1947).
[20] ZILBOORG and HENRY, *op. cit.*, p. 364.
[21] CHARCOT and MARIE, *op. cit.*, p. 635.
[22] ERIC J. DINGWALL, *Some Human Oddities* (London: Home and Van Thal, 1947).
GUILLAIN, *op. cit.*, p. 45.
[23] CHARCOT, *Lectures on the Diseases of the Nervous System* (London: New Sydenham Society, 1877), I, p. 249.
[24] SIR HORATIO B. DONKIN, 'Hysteria' in D. Hack Tuke, ed., *Dictionary of Psychological Medicine* (London: Churchill, 1892), I, p. 620.
[25] CHARCOT, *op. cit.*, pp. 229-230.
[26] *Loc. cit.*
[27] *Loc. cit.*
[28] JANET, *op. cit.*, pp. 272-277.
[29] *Loc. cit.*
[30] *Ibid.*, p. 198.
[31] CHARCOT, *op. cit.*, pp. 229-230.
[32] CHARCOT, *Clinical Lectures on the Diseases of the Nervous System*, III, p. 368.
[33] CHARCOT, *op. cit.*, p. 221.
[34] GUILLAIN, *op. cit.*, p. 155.
[35] *Ibid.*, p. 155.
[36] *Ibid.*, p. 146.
[37] CHARCOT and MARIE, *op. cit.*, p. 629.
[38] *Loc. cit.*
[39] SIGMUND FREUD, 'Charcot', *Collected Papers* (London: Hogarth Press, 1948), I, p. 21.
[40] FREUD, *An Autobiographical Study* (London: Hogarth Press, 1935), pp. 25-26.
[41] M. ROSENTHAL. *A Clinical Treatise on the Diseases of the Nervous System with a Preface by Professor Charcot* (London: 1881).
[42] JANET, *op. cit.*, pp. 10-11.
[43] CHARCOT and MARIE, *op. cit.*, p. 629.

237

[44] FREUD, *An Autobiographical Study*, pp. 41-42.
[45] FREUD, 'On the History of the Psycho-Analytical Movement', *Collected Papers* (London: Hogarth Press, 1948), I, pp. 294-295.
[46] *Ibid.*, p. 296.
[47] ZILBOORG and HENRY, *op. cit.*, p. 364.
[48] CHARCOT, *Lectures on the Diseases of the Nervous System*, I, p. 247.
[49] *Ibid.*, p. 275.
[50] *Ibid.*, p. 247.
[51] FREUD, 'Charcot', *Collected Papers*, I, pp. 18-19.

Chapter IV

[1] CLIFFORD E. ALLEN, *Modern Discoveries in Medical Psychology* (London: Pan Books, 1965).
[2] PIERRE JANET, *The Major Symptoms of Hysteria* (New York: Macmillan, 1907), pp. 11-12.
[3] AXEL MUNTHE, *The Story of San Michele* (London: Murray, 1936), p. 213.
[4] JEAN-MARTIN CHARCOT, *Clinical Lectures on the Diseases of the Nervous System* (London: New Sydenham Society), III, p. 319.
[5] J.-M. CHARCOT and PIERRE MARIE, 'Hysteria', in D. Hack Tuke, ed., *Dictionary of Psychological Medicine* (London: Churchill, 1892), I, p. 630.
[6] JANET, *op. cit.*, p. 16.
[7] CHARCOT, *Lectures on the Diseases of the Nervous System*, I, p. 230.
[8] *Loc. cit.*
[9] JANET, *op. cit.*, p. 125.
[10] *Ibid.*, pp. 162-163.
[11] *Ibid.*, pp. 148, 178.
[12] *Ibid.*, p. 174.
[13] *Loc. cit.*
[14] JANET, *Loc. cit.*
FREUD, 'Some points in a comparative study of organic and hysterical paralyses' *Collected Papers*, I, pp. 42-5.
[15] *Ibid.*, p. 42.
[16] FREUD, *An Autobiographical Study* (New York: Brentano, 1927), p. 22.
[17] JANET, *op. cit.*, pp. 157-158.
[18] FREUD, 'Some points in a comparative study of organic and hysterical paralyses,' p. 53.
[19] *Ibid.*, pp. 55-56.
[20] JANET, *op. cit.*, p. 175.
[21] *Loc. cit.*
[22] PETER HAYS, *New Horizons in Psychiatry* (London: Penguin Books, 1964).
M. RINKEL and J. C. B. DENBER, eds., *Chemical Concepts of Psychosis* (London: Peter Owen, 1961).
[23] CHARCOT, *Lectures on Senile and Chronic Diseases* (London: New Sydenham Society, 1881), I, p. 17.
[24] FREUD, *op. cit.*, p. 57.
[25] CHARCOT, *Clinical Lectures*, III, p. 222.
[26] *Loc. cit.*
[27] CHARCOT and MARIE, *op. cit.*, p. 639.

[28] CHARCOT, *Clinical Lectures*, III, p. 222.
[29] *Ibid.*, p. 245.
[30] *Ibid.*, p. 248.
[31] JANET, *op. cit.*, p. 141.
[32] *Loc. cit.*
[33] CHARCOT, *op. cit.*, p. 345.
[34] J. BREUER and S. FREUD, *Studies on Hysteria* (London: Hogarth Press, 1956), p. 213.
[35] *Ibid.*, p. 134.
[36] *Ibid.*, p. 213.
[37] *Ibid.*, p. 76n.
[38] CHARCOT, *op. cit.*, p. 305.
[39] ERNST KRETSCHMER, *Hysteria, Reflex and Instinct* (London: Peter Owen, 1961).
[40] *Ibid.*, p. 12.
[41] *Ibid.*, pp. 25-26.
[42] *Ibid.*, pp. 27-28.
[43] CHARCOT, *Lectures on Senile and Chronic Diseases*, I, p. 119.
[44] FREUD, 'Heredity and the Aetiology of the Neuroses,' *Collected Papers*, I.
[45] *Loc. cit.*, and 'Charcot,' *Collected Papers*, I.
[46] FREUD, 'Heredity and the Aetiology of the Neuroses'.
[47] STEVEN G. VANDENBERG, *Methods and Goals in Human Behaviour* (New York: Academic Press, 1965).
[48] F. W. BROWN, 'Heredity in the Psychoneuroses,' *Proceedings of the Royal Society of Medicine* (May 1942), XXV, pp. 785-790.
[49] E. SLATER, 'The Neurotic Constitution,' *Journal of Neurology and Psychiatry* (New Series), VI (1943), pp. 1-17.
[50] SIR RONALD A. FISHER, *The Genetical Theory of Natural Selection* (New York: Dover, 1958).
[51] CHARCOT and MARIE, 'Hysteria,' *Dictionary of Psychological Medicine,* p. 628.
[52] KRETSCHMER, *op. cit.*, pp. 50-54.
[53] CHARCOT and MARIE, *op. cit.*, p. 639.
[54] BREUER and FREUD, *op. cit.*, p. 232.
[55] CHARCOT, *Clinical Lectures*, III, p. 289.
[56] *Ibid.*, p. 290.
[57] FREUD, 'On the History of the Psychoanalytic Movement,' *Collected Papers* (London: Hogarth Press, 1948), I.
[58] CHARCOT, *op. cit.*, p. 29.
[59] J.-M. CHARCOT and PAUL RICHER, 'Note on certain facts of cerebral automatism. Suggestion by the muscular sense,' *Journal of Nervous and Mental Diseases,* (Jan. 1883), X.
[60] ALFRED BINET and CHARLES FÉRÉ, Le *Magnétisme Animal* (Paris: Alcan, 1887), pp. 76-77.
[61] CHARCOT, *op. cit.*, p. 291.
[62] *Ibid.*, pp. 292-293.
[63] *Ibid.*, pp. 305-306.
[64] BREUER and FREUD, *op. cit.*, pp. 15-16, 42-47.
FREUD, 'On the Psychical Mechanism of Hysterical Phenomena, *Collected Papers*, I, p. 39.
[65] CHARCOT, *op. cit.*, p. 372.

66 GEORGES GUILLAIN, *J.– M. Charcot. His Life—His Work* (London: Pitman Medical Publishing Company, 1959), p. 373.
67 FREUD, *An Autobiographical Study*, pp. 21-22.
67 FREUD, 'Charcot,' *Collected Papers*, I, p. 22.

Chapter V

1 ROBERT GRAVES, *The Greek Myths* (London: Penguin Books, 1955), I, p. 234.
2 PIERRE JANET, *Psychological Healing. A Historical and Clinical Study* New York: Macmillan, 1925), I, pp. 692-693.
3 CHARCOT, *Clinical Lectures on the Diseases of the Nervous System* (London: New Sydenham Society, 1889), III, p. 389
4 *Ibid.*, p. 405.
5 CHARCOT, *Lectures on Diseases of the Nervous System* (London: New Sydenham Society, 1889), I, p. 291.
6 CHARCOT, *Ibid.*, III, pp. 308n, 309n.
7 PIERRE JANET, *Psychological Healing*, I, pp. 326-327.
8 D. HACK TUKE, *Illustrations of the Influence of the Mind Upon the Body* (London: Churchill, 1884), p. 189.
9 CHARCOT, *op. cit.*, p. 307.
10 *Ibid.*, p. 308.
11 *Loc. cit.*
12 JANET, *op. cit.*, pp. 308-371.
13 ERNST KRETSCHMER, *Hysteria, Reflex and Instinct* (London: Peter Owen, 1956), pp. 110-134.
14 PIERRE JANET, *The Major Symptoms of Hysteria* (New York: Macmillan, 1907), p. 315.
15 CHARCOT, *op. cit.*, p. 309.
16 C. CHERVIN, *Béguiement considéré comme vice de prononciation* (Paris: 1867).
17 JANET, *Psychological Healing*, II, pp. 712-714.
18 CHARLES FÉRÉ, *Sensation et Mouvement* (Paris: Alcan, 1887).
F. LAGRANGE, *Les Mouvements méthodiques et la Mécanothérapie* (Paris: Alcan, 1889).
19 CHARCOT, *op. cit.*, p. 309.
20 FÉRÉ, *op. cit.*
21 JANET, *op. cit.*, p. 713.
22 G. GILLES DE LA TOURETTE, *Traité Clinique et Thérapeutique de l'Hystérie d'après l'Enseignement de la Salpêtrière* (Paris: Plon et Noimet, 1891-1899, 3 vols.).
23 FÉRÉ, *op. cit.*
24 CHARCOT, *op. cit.*, pp. 218-219.
25 *Ibid.*, pp. 78-79.
26 *Ibid.*, p. 80.
27 *Ibid.*, p. 82.
28 *Ibid.*, p. 167.
29 ARMAND BÉNET, *Procès verbal fait pour délivrer une fille possédée, Françoise Fontaine, à Louviers* (Paris: Progrès Médical, 1883).
30 CHARCOT, *op. cit.*, pp. 198-199.
31 *Ibid.*, p. 210.
32 *Loc. cit.*

240

[33] *Ibid.*, p. 218.
[34] JANET, *The Major Symptoms of Hysteria*, p. 232.
[35] CHARCOT, *op. cit.*, p. 212.
[36] *Ibid.*, p. 214.
[37] JANET, *op. cit.*, p. 234.
[38] D. M. BOURNEVILLE, *Science et Miracle. Louise Lateau ou la Stigmatisée belge* (Paris: 1875).
[39] WILLIAM IRVINE, *Apes, Angels and Victorians* (London: Weidenfeld and Nicholson, 1956).
[40] A. T. MYERS and F. W. H. MYERS, 'Mind, Faith-Cure and the Miracles of Lourdes.' *Proceedings of the Society for Psychical Research* 1893-4), pp. 160-209.
EMILE ZOLA, *Lourdes* (Paris: Fasquelle, 1903).
[41] CHARCOT, *La Foi qui Guérit* (Paris: Progrès Médical, 1897).
[42] L. B. CARRÉ DE MONTGERON, *La Vérité des Miracles Opérés par l'Intercession de M. de Pâris* (Utrecht, 1737).
[43] JANET, *Psychological Healing*, I, p. 26.
[44] E. T. WITHINGTON, The Asclepiadae and the Priests of Asclepius', in Charles Singer, ed., *Studies in the History and Method of Science* (1921), II, pp. 192-205.
[45] JOHN AUBREY, *Miscellanies upon Various Subjects* (London: 2nd ed. 1721), p. 130.
[46] *Loc. cit.*
[47] HACK TUKE, *op. cit.*, p. 223.
[48] CHARCOT, *op. cit.*, pp. 1-2.
[49] *Ibid.*, pp. 6-7.
[50] *Ibid.*, pp. 11-12.
[51] BOURNEVILLE, *op. cit.*
[52] GEORGES BERTRIN, *Lourdes, apparitions et guérisons* (Lourdes, 1905). *Histoire critique des èvènements de Lourdes* (Paris: Lecoffre, 1904).
[53] CHARCOT, *op. cit.*, p. 38.

Chapter VI

[1] ALFRED BINET and CHARLES FÉRÉ, *Animal Magnetism* (London: Kegan, Paul, Trench, 1887), p. 354.
[2] *Ibid.*, p(v).
[3] *Ibid.*, pp. 354-355.
[4] GEORGES GUILLAIN, *J.-M. Charcot. His Life—His Work* (London: Pitman Medical Publishing Company, 1959).
[5] OLIVER W. HOLMES, *Medical Essays* (Boston: Houghton Mifflin, 1883).
[6] CHARLES H. A. DESPINE, *De l'emploi du magnétisme animal et des eaux minérales dans le traitement des maladies nerveuses, etc.* (Paris: 1840.)
PIERRE JANET, *Psychological Healing* (New York: Macmillan, 1925), II, pp. 791-792.
[7] VICTOR BURQ, *Des origines de la metallotherapie: part qui doit être faite au magnétisme animal dans sa découverte: le Burgisme et le Perkinisme* (Paris: 1883).
[8] JANET, *op. cit.*, p. 795.
[9] GUILLAIN, *op. cit.*, p. 168.

[10] JANET, *op. cit.*, pp. 818-819.

[11] *Ibid.*, p. 822.

[12] HYPPOLYTE BERNHEIM, *De la suggestion dans l'état hypnotique et dans l'état de veille* (Paris: Doin, 1884); *De la suggestion et de ses applications à la thérapeutique* (Paris: Doin, 1886).

[13] SIGMUND FREUD, 'Hypnotism and Suggestion,' *Collected Papers* (London: Hogarth Press, 1948), V, p. 16.

[14] PIERRE JANET, *The Major Symptoms of Hysteria* (New York: Macmillan, 1907), pp. 298-299.

[15] FREUD, *op. cit.*, pp. 21-22.

[16] *Ibid.*

[17] JANET, *op. cit.*, p. 301.

[18] *Loc. cit.*

[19] PAUL A. SOLLIER, *Genèse et nature de l'hystérie, recherches cliniques et expérimentales de psycho-physiologie* (Paris: 1897).

[20] JANET, *Psychological Healing*, II, p. 822.

[21] *Ibid.*, p. 798.

[22] *Ibid.*, p. 799.

[23] *Ibid.*, pp. 799-800.

[24] *Ibid.*, pp. 789-790.

[25] JANET, *The Major Symptoms of Hysteria*, p. 60.

[26] PIERRE JANET, 'Autobiography' in C. Murchison, ed., *A History of Psychology in Autobiography* (Worcester, Mass: Clark University Press, 1930), p. 124.

[27] *Ibid*, p. 125.

[28] GEORGES GUINON, *Clinique des Maladies du Système Nerveux. M. le Professeur Charcot* (Paris: Progrès Médical, Barbe, 1893), II.

[29] PIERRE JANET, *The Mental State of Hystericals, with a Preface by Professor J.-M. Charcot* (New York: Putnam, 1901).

[30] GREGORY ZILBOORG and G. W. HENRY, *A History of Medical Psychology* (New York: Norton, 1941), p. 376.

[31] SIGMUND FREUD, 'Charcot,' *Collected Papers* (London: Hogarth Press, 1948), I, p. 16.

[32] JANET, *op. cit.*, p. 334.

[33] JANET, *Psychological Healing*, II, pp. 794-795.

[34] CHARCOT, *Clinical Lectures on the Diseases of the Nervous System* (London: New Sydenham Society, 1889), III, p. 198.

[35] JANET, *op. cit.*, II, p. 214.

[36] *Ibid.*, pp. 826-827.

[37] PIERRE JANET, *Psychological Healing*, I, pp. 326-327.

[38] EILEEN J. GARRETT, 'Dynamics of Healing,' *Proceedings of Four Conferences of Parapsychological Studies* (New York: Parapsychology Foundation, Inc., 1957), pp. 75-76.

[39] FREDERICK W. H. MYERS, *Human Personality and its Survival of Bodily Death* (London: Longmans Green, 1904).

[40] EMILIO SERVADIO, *Unconscious and Paranormal Factors in Healing and Recovery*—15th F. W. H. Myers Memorial Lecture (London: Society for Psychical Research, 1963).

[41] GARRETT, *op. cit.*, p. 74.

[42] JANET, *The Mental State of Hystericals*, pp. 151-155.

Chapter VII

[1] ALFRED BINET and CHARLES FÉRÉ, *Animal Magnetism* (London: Kegan, Paul, Trench, 1887), p. 8.
[2] *Ibid.*, p. 11.
[3] PIERRE JANET, *The Mental State of Hystericals* (New York: Putnam, 1901), p. 152.
[4] BINET and FÉRÉ, *op cit.*, p. 18.
[5] ERIC J. DINGWALL, ed., *Abnormal Hypnotic Phenomena: A Survey of Nineteenth-Century Cases* (London: Churchill, 1967-8).
[6] JANET, *op. cit.*, p. 444.
FREDERICK W. H. MYERS, *Human Personality* (London: Longmans Green, 1904).
[7] JANET, *op. cit.*, p. 445.
[8] A. J. F. BERTRAND, *Traité du somnambulisme et des différentes modifications qu'il présente* (Paris: 1823).
[9] J. C. DE FARIA, *De la cause du sommeil lucide* (Paris: 1819).
[10] BINET and FÉRÉ, *op. cit.*, p. 33.
[11] *Ibid.*, p. 77.
[12] F. J. NOIZET, *Mémoire sur le somnambulisme et le magnétisme animal* (Paris: Plon, 1854).
[13] JAMES BRAID, *Neurypnology or the Rationale of Nervous Sleep Considered in Relation to Animal Magnetism* (London: Churchill, 1843).
[14] BERTRAND, *op. cit.*
J. P. F. DELEUZE, *Histoire critique du magnétisme animal*, 2 vols. (Paris: 1813).
J. DU POTET DE SENNEVOY, *Manuel de l'étuliant magnétiseur de nouvelle instruction practique du magnétisme* (Paris: Baillière, 1846).
L. J. J. CHARPIGNON, *Physiologie, médecine et métaphysique du magnétisme* (Paris: Baillière, 1848).
[15] AMBROISE A. LIÉBEAULT, *Du sommeil et des états analogues considérés surtout au point de vue de l'action morale sur le physique* (Nancy and Paris: 1866).
[16] JAMES M. BRAMWELL, *Hypnotism, its History, Practice and Theory* (Philadelphia: Lippincott, 1938), p. 31.
[17] FREDERICK W. H. MYERS, *Human Personality* (London: Longmans Green, 1904).
[18] E. MESNET, *De l'automatisme de mémoire et du souvenir dans le somnambulisme pathologique; considérations médicolégales* (Paris: 1874).
[19] PIERRE JANET, *Psychological Healing* (New York: Macmillan, 1925), I, p. 167.

Chapter VIII

[1] CHARCOT, *Oeuvres Complètes* (Paris: Progrès Médical, 1890), IX.
[2] *Loc. cit.*
[3] D. M. BOURNEVILLE and P. REGNARD, *L'Iconographie Photographique de la Salpêtrière*, 3 vols. (Paris: Delahaye, 1877-1882).
[4] P. LADAME, *La Névrose hypnotique* (Paris: Sandoz and Fischbacker, 1881).

[5] A. T. MYERS, 'History of Hypnotism,' in D. Hack Tuke, ed., *Dictionary of Psychological Medicine* (London: Churchill, 1892).

[6] ALFRED BINET, *The Psychology of Reasoning based on Experimental Research in Hypnosis* (London: Kegan, Paul, Trench, Trübner, 1899), p. 59.

ALFRED BINET and CHARLES FÉRÉ, *Animal Magnetism* (London: Kegan Paul, Trench, Trübner, 1887), p. 230.

[7] FREDERICK W. H. MYERS, *Human Personality* (New York: Longmans Green, 1904), I, p. 447.

[8] BINET, *op. cit.*, pp. 59-60.

[9] J. LIÉGEOIS, *De la Suggestion et du Somnambulisme dans leurs rapports avec la Jurisprudence et la Médecine Légale* (Paris: Doin, 1889).

[10] BINET and FÉRÉ, *op. cit.*, p. 230.

[11] *Loc. cit.*

[12] LIÉGEOIS, *op. cit.*

[13] C. LLOYD TUCKEY, *Treatment by Hypnotism and Suggestion* (London: Bailliere, Tyndall and Cox, 1900), pp. 402-403.

[14] HIPPOLYTE BERNHEIM, *De la suggestion dans l'état hypnotique et dans l'état de veille* (Paris: Doin, 1886); *De la suggestion et ses applications à la thérapeutique* (Paris: Doin, 1886).

LIÉGEOIS, *op. cit.*

[15] GEORGES GILLES DE LA TOURETTE, *L'Hypnotisme et les états analogues au point de vue médico-légal*, with a Preface by Professor Brouardel (Paris: Doin, 1887).

[16] PIERRE JANET, *Psychological Healing* (New York: Macmillan, 1925), I, p. 184.

[17] F. W. H. MYERS, *op. cit.*, I, pp. 447-448.

[18] J.-M. CHARCOT and G. GILLES DE LA TOURETTE, 'Hypnotism in the Hysterical,' in D. Hack Tuke, ed., *Dictionary of Psychological Medicine* (London: Churchill, 1891), I, p. 606.

[19] *Loc. cit.*

[20] JANET, *op. cit.*, I, p. 296.

[21] P. BRIQUET, *Traité clinique et thérapeutique de l'hystérie* (Paris: 1859).

[22] LLOYD TUCKEY, *op. cit.*, p. 123.

[23] *Loc. cit.*

[24] BINET and FÉRÉ, *op. cit.*, pp. 88-94.

JANET, *op. cit.*, pp. 298-300.

[25] CHARCOT, *Oeuvres Complètes* (Paris: Delahaye et Lecrosnier, 1885-90), IV.

[26] GEORGES GUILLAIN, *J.-M. Charcot. His Life—His Work* (London: Pitman Medical Publishing Company, 1959), pp. 8-9.

[27] *Ibid.* p. 167.

[28] AXEL MUNTHE, *The Story of San Michele* (London: Murray, 1936), p. 220.

[29] GUILLAIN, *op. cit.*, p. 28.

[30] *Ibid.*, p. 17.

[31] *Ibid.*, p. 61.

[32] *Ibid.*, p. 19.

[33] JANET, *op. cit.*, p. 170.

[34] GUILLAIN, *op. cit.*, p. 55.

[35] SIGMUND FREUD, 'Charcot,' *Collected Papers* (London: Hogarth Press, 1948), I, p. 17.

[36] GEORGES GUINON, *Clinique des Maladies du Système Nerveux. M. le Professeur Charcot* (Paris: Progrès Médical, 1893), II.
[37] FREUD, *op. cit.*, p. 18.
[38] MUNTHE, *op. cit.*, pp. 214, 219.
[39] GUILLAIN, *op. cit.*, p. 63.
[40] J.-M. CHARCOT and PIERRE MARIE, 'Hysteria,' in D. Hack Tuke, ed., *Dictionary of Psychological Medicine* (London: Churchill, 1891), I, p. 640.
[41] JANET, *op. cit.*, p. 359.
[42] S. FREUD, *An Autobiographical Study* (New York: Brentano, 1927), p. 48.
[43] JANET, *op. cit.*, pp. 314-315.
[44] MUNTHE, *op. cit.*, p. 219.
[45] MUNTHE, *op. cit.*, pp. 220-226.
GUSTAF MUNTHE and G. VEXKULL, *The Story of Axel Munthe* (London: Murray, 1953).
[46] BERNHEIM, *op. cit.* (1884).
[47] JANET, *op. cit.*, p. 193.
[48] *Ibid.*, pp. 200-201.
[49] GUILLAIN, *op. cit.*, p. 171.
[50] JANET, *op. cit.*, p. 191.
DU POTET DE SENNEVOY, *op. cit.*
[51] JANET, *op. cit.*, p. 35.
[52] *Ibid.*, pp. 187-190.
F. W. H. MYERS, *op. cit.*
[53] JANET, *op. cit.*, p. 192.

Chapter IX

[1] ALAN R. G. OWEN, *Can We Explain The Poltergeist?* (New York: Helix Press-Garrett Publications, 1964).
ARMAND BÉNET, *Procès Verbal, fait pour délivrer une fille possédée, Françoise Fontaine, à Louviers.* Intro. B. de Moray (Paris: Progrès Médical, 1883).
[2] A. R. G. OWEN, 'Brownie, Incubus and Poltergeist,' *International Journal of Parapsychology* (1964), VI, pp. 455-472.
M. WILLIAMS, 'The Poltergeist Man,' *International Journal of Parapsychology* (1964), VI, pp. 423-454.
[3] D. M. BOURNEVILLE, *La Possession de Jeanne Fery de Mans, 1584* (Paris: Progrès Médical, 1897).
[4] J.-M. CHARCOT, *La Foi qui guérit* (Paris: Progrès Médical, 1897).
[5] D. M. BOURNEVILLE, *Science et Miracle. Louise Lateau ou la Stigmatisée belge* (Paris: 1875).
[6] CHARCOT, *Loc. cit.*
[7] FREDERICK W. H. MYERS, *Human Personality* (New York: Longmans Green, 1904), I, p. 498.
[8] J.-M. CHARCOT and P. MARIE, 'Hysteria,' in D. Hack Tuke, ed., *Dictionary of Psychological Medicine* (London: Churchill, 1892), I, p. 637.
[9] AXEL MUNTHE, *The Story of San Michele* (London: Murray, 1936), p. 219.

[10] PIERRE JANET, 'Autobiography,' in C. Murchison, ed., *A History of Psychology in Autobiography* (Worcester, Mass.: Clark University Press, 1930), I, p. 125.
[11] MYERS, *op. cit.*, I, p. 172.
[12] JANET, *op. cit.*
[13] CLAPARÈDE, 'Autobiography' in C. Murchison, ed., *op. cit.*, pp. 63-97.
[14] GEORGES GUILLAIN, *J.-M. Charcot. His Life—His Work* (London: Pitman Medical Publishing Company, 1959), p. 7.
[15] CLAPARÈDE, *op. cit.*, p. 72.

Chapter X

[1] SIGMUND FREUD 'Charcot,' *Collected Papers* (London: Hogarth Press, 1948), I, p. 9.
[2] MARTHE OULIÉ, *Charcot and the Antarctic* (London: Murray, 1938), p. 3.
[3] SACHEVERELL SITWELL, *La Vie Parisienne* (London: Faber, 1937).
[4] *Ibid.*
[5] S. KRACAUER, *Offenbach and the Paris of His Time* (London: Constable, 1937).
[6] OULIÉ, *op. cit.*, p. 5.
[7] GREGORY ZILBOORG and G. W. HENRY, *A History of Medical Psychology* (New York: Norton, 1941), p. 370.
[8] J.-M. CHARCOT, *Lectures on Senile and Chronic Diseases* (London: New Sydenham Society, 1881), p. 22.
[9] *Loc. cit.*
[10] FREUD, *op. cit.*, p. 22.
[11] LOUIS GALLET, *Guerre et commune impression d'un hospitalier* (Paris: Calmann-Lévy, 1898).
GEORGES GUILLAIN, *J.-M. Charcot. His Life—His Work* (London: Pitman Medical Publishing Company, 1959), p. 12.
[12] AXEL MUNTHE, *The Story of San Michele* (London: Murray, 1936), p. 206.
[13] FREUD, *op. cit.*, pp. 14-15.
[14] OULIÉ, *op. cit.*, p. 22.
[15] FREUD, *op. cit.*, p. 16.
[16] PIERRE JANET, *The Mental State of Hystericals* (New York: Putnam, 1901).
[17] GUILLAIN, *op. cit.*, p. 35.
[18] GUILLAIN, *op. cit.*

APPENDIX

Bibliothèque Diabolique (Collection Bourneville)

(Paris: Aux Bureaux du *Progrès Médical.*)

1882 : M. D. BOURNEVILLE et E. TEINTURIER : Le Sabbat des Sorciers.

1883 : A. BENET : *Procès verbal fait pour delivrer une fille possédée, Françoise Fontaine, à Louviers.* With an Introduction by B. de Moray.

1885 : J. WEIER : *Histoires, disputes et discours* and *Two Dialogues* by Thomas Erastus. With a Preface by D. M. Bourneville, and a biography of Weier by L. Axenfeld. 2 vols.

1886 : D. M. BOURNEVILLE : *La possession de Jeanne Fery de Mans* (1584).

1886 : G. G. LEGUE, et G. GILLES DE LA TOURETTE : *Sœur Jeanne des Anges, Supérieure des Ursulines de Loudun—Autobiographie d'une hystérique possédee.* With a Preface by Professor Charcot.

1888 : P. LADAME : *Procès Criminal de la dernière sorcière brûlée à Genève le 6 avril 1652.*

1895 : S. GARNIER : *Barbe Buvée, en religion Sœur Sainte-Colombe, et la prétendue possession des Ursulines d'Auxonne* (1658-1663). With a Preface by D. M. Bourneville.

1897 J.-M. CHARCOT, *La Foi qui Guérit.* With a Preface by D. M. Bourneville.

A

A, Mlle, 76, 77
Abasia, 68, 73
Abulia, 129
Academy of Sciences, 185
Achromatopsia, 67
    See also Visual Disturbances
Aesculapius, 17, 141
Aesthesiogens, 152–168, 173
Alleviative treatment, 42
Alphand, 219
Amyotrophic lateral sclerosis, 40
Anesthesias, 62, 66, 67, 70, 71, 73–5,
    78, 79, 81, 83, 86–123, 139, 169
    See also Hysteria
Anselin, Adèle, 52
Aphasia, 51, 193
Aretaeus, 58
Arthralgia, 67
Asclepiades, 23
Astasia, 68, 73
Aubrey, John, 141
Autosuggestion, 99, 102, 105, 146,
    155–157, 191
Azam, Dr, 104, 116, 159, 180, 183,
    185, 190

B

Babinski, 45, 71, 90, 108, 205
Bailly, 174
Bamberg, 80
Bar., Alphonsine, 185, 186, 194, 211
Baragnon, 209
Beaujon Hospital, 184
Beaunis, 182
Berna, 178
Bernard, Claude, 42
Bernheim, Hippolyte, 139, 140, 148,
    154, 156, 165, 167, 182, 189, 197,
    200, 201, 206–208
Bertrand, Dr, 177, 179, 180, 194
Bertrin, 145
Bicêtre, 26
Bichat, 21
Binet, Alfred, 148, 149, 164, 187–
    189, 195

Bismarck, 223, 224
Bla., 193
Bottard, Mlle, 137–228
Bottey, 209
Bouchard, Charles, 41, 52, 164
Bourneville, Désiré Magloire, 69, 71,
    72, 140, 147, 152, 153, 164, 183,
    185, 186, 209, 212, 215, 223
Boyle, Robert, 27
Brachet, 60
Braid, James, 151, 179, 180, 183,
    195
Bramwell, 164, 181
Bravais, 53
Breuer, 82, 102–105, 111, 112, 120,
    205
Briquet, Pierre, 60, 79, 80, 83, 108,
    192
Brissaud, 51, 130, 183, 186, 199
Broca, Paul, 38, 50, 52, 164, 180,
    183, 184, 209
Brodie, Sir Benjamin, 60, 96, 112
Brouardel, Professor, 78, 82, 147,
    188, 215
Brouillet, 71
Brown, 110
Burq, Dr Victor, 98, 151, 152, 166,
    168, 184

C

Cabanis, 157
Cartaz, Dr, 203
Castiglioni, 69
Catalepsy, 177, 184–211
Catatonia, Kahlbaum's, 58
Celsus, 25
Cephalgia, 67
Cerebral localization, 51, 53
Chambard, 183
Charcot, Jean, 68, 221, 228, 231,
    232, 234
Charcot, Jean-Martin
    birth, 29
    Chair of Diseases of the Nervous
        System, 47, 55, 61
    Chef de Clinique, 32

chief of medical services, 33
death, 233
doctoral thesis, 31
early education, 30
Externat des Hôpitaux, 30
founder of neurology, 29–54
internship, 30, 31
junior consultant, 32
lecture courses, 45, 47
medical degree, 30
Médecin des Hôpitaux, 32, 33
medical training, 30
neurological studies, 29
private practice, 32
Professeur Agrégé, 33
Professeur de Chaire, 47
Professor of Pathological Anat-
  omy, 45, 46, 225
supernatural, 212–16
  See also Hysteria, Hypnosis,
  Neuroses, Saltpêtrière
Charcot, Jeanne, 221, 231
Charcot, Madame, 220, 221, 225–7,
  231
Charetie, Jules, 187
Charpignon, 175, 180
Chavigny, Professor, 78
Chermitte, Professor, 79
Chervin, Claudius, 129, 130
Chorea, 29, 55, 67, 69
Chrobak, 82
Clairvoyant diagnosis, 178
Claparède, 215, 216
Clinico-anatomical method, 38, 51
Cloquet, 178
Coirin, Louise, 144, 145, 212
Comte, 215
Congress of Psychology, 50
Contractures, 67, 75, 76, 88, 89,
  139, 145
  See also Hysteria
Convulsionnaires, 70, 71, 84, 135
Convulsive attacks, 63, 64
Conway, Lady, 171
Corneil, 44
Croesus, 124
Cruveilhier, 28, 37

D
d'Albret, Jeanne, 140
Daquin, Joseph, 27
d'Artois, Comte, 172
Daudet, Alphonse, 229
Daudet, Léon, 48, 232
Darwin, Charles, 110, 116
De Baïssas, 210
Debove, Professor, 46, 199, 233
de Garnay, Hébert, 209

Dejerine, 216
de La Mettrie, 21
Delasiauve, Dr, 57
de la Tourette, Gilles, 108, 130,
  132, 133, 145, 169, 189, 192,
  195
Deleuze, 175, 180
Demarquay, 181, 183
de Montgeron, Carré, 141, 144
De Moray, 212
de Pâris, François, 70, 144
de Puyfontaine, Marquis, 211
de Puységur, Armand, 117, 174,
  175, 190
d'Eslon, Charles, 172, 174
Dom Pedro, 230
Donkin, Sir Horatio, 72
Dreyfus, Alfred, 215
Dubois, Dr, 178
Duchenne de Boulogne, Guillaume,
  38, 60, 116
Dum., 98, 117, 152
Dumont, 182
Dumontpallier, 152, 157, 190, 209
Du Potet de Sennevoy, 160, 175,
  177, 178, 180, 209–211
Durand de Gros, 181
Durvis, Augustine Victoire,
  see Madame Charcot
Durvis, Marie, 220, 230
du Saulle, 60
du Tranchay, Louise, 25

E
Epilepsy, 23, 24, 29, 53, 55, 57,
  60, 87
Erb, 108
Esdaille, 178
Esquirol, 28
Estelle, 159
Etch., Justine, 100, 102, 111, 149
Eugénie, Mlle, 176, 177

F
Faith healing, 71, 88, 124–146, 148,
  149, 164, 165, 167
Faith That Heals, 141, 142
Falguière, 234
Faria, Abbé, 135, 177, 192
Félida X, 104, 116, 159, 180
Féré, 95, 101, 130, 131, 147–149,
  164, 188, 189, 195
Fery, Jeanne, 212
Finger-tip reading, 178
Fisher, 111
Flourens, 51
Flournoy, 215

Fludd, Robert, 170
Follin, 180, 183
Fontaine, Françoise, 134, 212
Formes frustes, 66, 194
Fould, 218
Fournier, 108
Fowler, 145
Franklin, Benjamin, 172, 174
Frenkel, 130
Freud, 29, 35, 36, 47, 48, 53, 56,
    62, 65, 69, 77, 80–82, 84, 92–94,
    96, 102–105, 108, 109, 114, 120,
    122, 123, 154, 155, 203–205, 223
Functional lesions, 93, 94, 95

G
Galen, 19, 20, 23, 24, 59
Gallet, Louis, 225
Galton, 110
Gambetta, 47, 222, 224, 230, 231
Garrett, Eileen, 166, 167
Garrod, 107
Gasteralgia, 67
Gellé, 152
Georget, 177
Gesterlin, Fräulein, 171
Gibert, Dr, 160, 210
Giraud-Teulon, 181, 183
Glaiz., Louise, 185, 186, 194, 211
Globus hystericus, 63, 66
Gombault, 43
Goncourt, 204
Grande attaque, 66
Graves, Robert, 223
Greatrakes, Valentine, 171
Greuz., 118–120, 126
Guérineau, 180
Guillain, Georges, 29, 40, 41, 58,
    122, 150, 153, 183, 202, 211
Guillotin, Dr, 174
Guinon, Georges, 58, 108, 122, 130,
    161, 202, 227, 229
Gull, Sir William, 137

H
Hablon, Marie, 161
Hall, Stanley, 50
Hallucination, 187, 188
Haussmann, Baron, 219
Hecquet, 71, 84
Hélène, 78
Heidenhain, 209
Hell, Maximilian, 171
Hendry, Arthur, 234
Herodotus, 124
Hippocrates, 18, 58, 60
Holmes, Oliver Wendell, 151
Hopkins, Matthew, 70

Hospice Général, 26
Hôtel-Dieu, 177
Hüchel, 154
Hugo, Victor, 222
Hume, David, 49
Husson Commission, 178
Husson, Dr, 177, 178, 211
Huxley, Aldous, 25
Huxley, Thomas, 140
Hyoscine, 42
Hypnosis, 113–123, 161, 170–211
Hypochondria, 56
Hysteria, 55, 56–59, 61, 63, 65–67,
    69, 72–75, 78, 79, 81, 83–123
    causes of, 85–123
    hereditary basis, 107, 108
    male, 59, 79, 82, 90
    predisposition, 110–112
    sexual drives, 81–84

I
Idée fixe, 99
Ignotus, 198, 200
Iphiclus, 124
Ischuria, 72, 73

J
Jackson, Hughlings, 53
James, William, 49, 50
Janet, Jules, 89, 157, 159, 190,
    210, 230
Janet, Paul, 160, 161
Janet, Pierre, 29, 49, 59, 62, 65,
    66, 73–75, 81, 85, 88, 93–95, 99,
    100, 108, 111, 124, 129, 139,
    141, 153–162, 165, 168, 173, 174,
    176, 183, 186, 190, 191, 195, 205,
    206, 209–211, 213
Jansen, 70
Joffroy, 43, 44, 122
Jung, Carl, 65, 69, 115

K
Katharina, 102, 103
Kingsbury, Dr, 189
Koch, Emil, 107
Kretschmer, 105, 129

L
Lacordaire, 179
Ladame, 157, 185
Laennec, 151
Lafontaine, 175, 179
Lagrange, 100
Landouzy, 60
La Pitié, 89, 160
Lasègue, 137, 139, 147, 184, 195
Lashley, 51

Lateau, Louise, 145, 212, 213
Lavoisier, 174
Le Log., 100, 124
Lenoble, Abbé, 151
Léonie, 160, 210, 213
Lepois, Charles, 59, 79
Ler., 100, 103
Lethargy, 184–211
Levallois, 22
Leyden, 130
Liébeault, 164, 181–183, 200, 204
Liégeois, 182, 187–189
Liouville, Dr, 230
Liouville, Jacques, 230
Lister, 86
Locomotor ataxia, 40
    See also Tabes dorsalis
Lombroso, 50
Londe, 186, 187
Lourdes, 140–145
Luys, Dr, 165, 206
Lys., 100, 101

M
Magendie, 22, 28
Magnetic Societies, 175
Magnetism, 170–183
Magnets, 147–169
Magnin, 209
Marie, Pierre, 35, 52, 62, 79, 99,
    121, 125, 164, 229
Massage, 132, 133
Maxwell, William, 170, 171
Mazarin, Cardinal, 26
Medicine, history of
    ancient, 15
    early 19th century, 22
    Egyptian, 16
    folk, 15
    Greek, 17, 23
    medieval, 25
Meige, Henri, 130
Mendel, Gregor, 111
Meningitis, syphilitic, 90
Mental elaboration, 102, 103, 144,
    164
Mesl., 119, 120
Mesmer, Franz Anton, 135, 151,
    170–174, 177, 192
    See also Hypnotism, Magnetism
Mesnet, 183
Metallotherapy, 98, 147–169
Meynert, 57, 80
More, Dr Henry, 42
Morel, 177
Morin, 175
Multiple sclerosis, 39

Munthe, Axel, 35, 41, 42, 56, 86,
    198, 203, 205, 206, 213, 226
Munthe, Gustaf, 206
Mutism, 77, 78, 130
Myers, A. T., 213
Myers, F. W. H., 166, 213, 214

N
Napoleon, Louis, 219, 221, 222, 224
Naquet, 230
Nervous shock, 104
Neurasthenia, 56
Neurology, 29, 37
    See also Charcot, Jean-Martin
Neuroses, 55–84, 90
    See also Freud, Jung
Neurosurgery, 86
Nightingale, Florence, 137
Noizet, General, 179, 192

O
Oedema, 145
Offenbach, 223
Oudet, Dr, 178
Oulié, Marthe, 232
Ovaralgia, 67, 70, 71

P
Paget, Sir James, 40
Paracelsus, 80, 170
Paradis, Fräulein, 172
Paralyses, 62, 67, 68, 85–123, 145
    See also Faith healing, Hysteria
Parguin, Louise, 127
Pariset, 28
Parkinson's disease, 39
Pasteur, Louis, 107, 230, 233
Perkins, 151
Perrier, Dr, 160, 175, 210
Pététin, 209
Petulle, Professor, 45
Phillips, 181
Pin., 89, 91, 97, 119, 120, 124,
    126, 128, 131, 132
Pinel, Philippe, 27, 28, 37, 84
Pinfield, 51
Pirandello, 204
Pitres, 53, 130, 153, 209
Plato, 20
Poliomyelitis, 44
Porcz., 91, 97, 119, 120, 126, 128,
    131, 132
Potain, Professor, 30, 233
Powilewicz, Dr, 160, 176
Praxis Medica, 59
Prévost, 44
Psellus, Michael, 24
Puel, 209

R
Railway spine, 78, 104
Rayer, 32, 38, 72, 198, 215, 217–219
Raymond, Professor, 130
Reade, Charles, 25
Reeducation therapy, 129, 131, 132, 138, 155
Reflex hyperexcitability, 96–98, 155, 161
Régnard, Paul, 69, 153, 185
Reynolds, Russell, 112, 113
Ribot, Théodule, 49, 161, 230
Richard, Laurent, 220, 221, 224
Richer, Paul, 68, 69, 115, 130, 143, 152, 183, 185, 186, 188, 201
Richet, Charles, 49, 160, 176, 183, 184, 213, 214, 230
Rig., 97
Rist, Dr, 46
Rivière, Lazare, 59
Rosenthal, 80
Roulier, Joséphine, 73
Ruault, 186
Rush, Benjamin, 25

S
St Dympna, 25
Saint Louis, 139
Saint Médard,135
St Radegonde, 143
St Vincent de Paul, 26, 137
Salmon, Thomas, 25
Saltpêtrière, 14, 23, 25–28, 46, 184, 211
Schizophrenia, 58, 65, 95
Schneider, Hortense, 224
School of Nancy, 188
Scipion, 26
Sclerosis, cerebral, 96
Sclerosis, spinal, 96
Scott, Samuel, 142
Seglar, 130
Semmelweis, 86
Seppili, 209
Servadio, Emilio, 167
Sidgwick, 214
Silver nitrate, 42
Slater, 110
Societé de Biologie, 184
Society of Harmony, 175, 180
Society of Physiological Psychology, 49, 160
Sollier, 157, 173, 190
Somnambulism, 58, 66, 103, 104,
158, 159,-161, 175, 184–211
See also Hypnosis
Soubirous, Bernadette, 140
Souques, Dr, 199
Straus, 233
Stupor, 105
Substitution, 156, 157
Suggestion, 129, 166, 167, 176, 177, 201
Sydenham, 56, 145

T
Tabes dorsalis, 40, 41, 89, 90, 108
Tamburini, 209
Teste, 209
Tetanus, 29
Thiers, 224
Ticks, 67, 77, 130, 131
Tillaux, Professor, 86
Todd, 92
Tostan, 177
Transfer, 152, 153, 155, 162
Trousseau, 52, 151
Tuke, Hack, 25, 43, 62, 63, 112, 127, 142, 186, 191, 197
Twilight states, 105

V
Vallery-Radot, 216, 233
van Helmont, 170, 171
Velpeau, 180
Vesalius, 20
Vigouroux, Romain, 152, 153, 165
Virchow, 212, 223
Visual disturbances, 74, 75, 78, 100, 134
Vitalism, 21
von N. Emmy, 104
von Ranke, Heinrich, 223
Vulpian, Édmé-Félix, 30, 33, 34, 37–39, 44, 45, 181, 183, 230

W
Waldeck-Rousseau, 215, 230
Weier, Johann, 71
Weismann, 110
Weiss, Madame, 189
Wittman, Blanche, 186–190, 194, 205, 210, 211
Wundt, 50

Z
Zilboorg, Gregory, 69, 83, 162, 222
Zola, Emile, 140